Also by Michael T. Murray

The Encyclopedia of Healing Foods

The Encyclopedia of Natural Medicine

The Complete Book of Juicing

What the Drug Companies Won't Tell You and Your Doctor Doesn't Know

How to Prevent and Treat Cancer with Natural Medicine

How to Prevent and Treat Diabetes with Natural Medicine

Dr. Murray's Total Body Tune-Up

The Pill Book Guide to Natural Medicine

THE MAGIC OF FOOD

The
MAGIC
of
FOOD

Live Longer and Healthier—and Lose Weight—
with the Synergetic Diet

Michael T. Murray, ND

ATRIA PAPERBACK
New York   London   Toronto   Sydney   New Delhi

ATRIA
PAPERBACK

An Imprint of Simon & Schuster, Inc.
1230 Avenue of the Americas
New York, NY 10020

First Atria paperback edition July 2018

ATRIA PAPERBACK and colophon are trademarks of Simon & Schuster, Inc.

For information about special discounts for bulk purchases, please contact Simon & Schuster Special Sales at 1-866-506-1949 or business@simonandschuster.com.

The Simon & Schuster Speakers Bureau can bring authors to your live event. For more information or to book an event, contact the Simon & Schuster Speakers Bureau at 1-866-248-3049 or visit our website at www.simonspeakers.com.

Interior design by Amy Trombat

Manufactured in the United States of America

10 9 8 7 6 5 4 3 2 1

Library of Congress Cataloging-in-Publication Data
Names: Murray, Michael T., author.
Title: The magic of food : live longer and healthier—and lose weight—with
   the synergetic diet / Michael T. Murray, N.D.
Description: First Atria Books hardcover edition. | New York : Atria Books,
   2017. | Includes bibliographical references and index.
Identifiers: LCCN 2017009978 (print) | LCCN 2017023063 (ebook)
Subjects: LCSH: Nutrition. | Medicine, Preventive. | Self-care, Health. |
   BISAC: HEALTH & FITNESS / Nutrition. | HEALTH & FITNESS / Naturopathy. |
   HEALTH & FITNESS / Alternative Therapies.
Classification: LCC RA784 (ebook) | LCC RA784.M86 2017 (print) | DDC
   613.2—dc23
LC record available at https://lccn.loc.gov/2017009978

ISBN 978-1-4516-6297-9
ISBN 978-1-4516-6298-6 (pbk)
ISBN 978-1-4516-6299-3 (ebook)

To my sister, Melanie, for a lifetime of love and support, especially during our early and later years. Your heart is the biggest and most tender that I have known. Thank you for always being there for me. I love and appreciate you.

Contents

Preface

FOOD HAS ALWAYS BEEN MAGICAL TO ME. FOOD NOURISHES, HEALS, COMFORTS, inspires, and brings us joy throughout our lives. There's nothing else that has this kind of power. Even after a lifetime of studying food and nutrition, I am still awed by the inherent magic of nature and the food that she gives us. Now a new era of food awareness is emerging; people are concerned as much about healthfulness and diversity of foods as they are about flavor. Healthier foods are now being served everywhere from high-end white-tablecloth restaurants to fast-food chains, from airport concessions to mall food courts. Convenience stores and mainstream grocery stores are also improving the quality of food they stock.

With the epidemic of obesity, diabetes, cancer, and other diet-related diseases exploding, not just in the United States but also worldwide, improvements in the quality of food we eat cannot happen soon enough. I believe that food is going to become a primary form of medicine, even as eating good food remains one of life's great pleasures. We will be able to tailor what we eat to our unique dietary requirements and health goals and still please our palates.

Through *The Magic of Food*, my goal is to stir your passion for healthful eating and inspire you to make the right choices for your well-being. I have packed *The Magic of Food* with sound, medically based information to lead you on a journey on which you will discover the remarkable ways in which food can have a magical, yet real, impact on your body, mind, and health.

One of the major concepts in *The Magic of Food* is "synergetics." Simply put, synergetics is how different foods and dietary factors work together to achieve a positive effect greater than the sum of each individual factor. So, in this case 1 + 1 + 1 does not equal 3 but something much greater.

The Magic of Food

- Explains the principles of the world's healthiest diets and latest science of nutrition
- Clarifies the revolutionary application of the effects of food on genetic expression
- Explains why phytochemicals are the "vitamins" of the twenty-first century and reveals my seven favorite superfoods
- Details which foods to eat as well as which ones to avoid for your health and total well-being
- Offers advice on which supplements to take and how much of them when you can't get all of your nutrition from food
- Includes recipes and a meal plan for the Synergetic Diet

The Magic of Food brings together the latest scientific information about how specific foods work together to make you healthier and still give you the satisfaction and delight that you expect from the food you eat.

In good health,

Michael T. Murray, ND
DoctorMurray.com

1

You Are What You Eat

In the early 1900s, Henry Lindlahr, MD, helped lay the groundwork for what became known as naturopathic medicine—medicine that emphasizes prevention and treatment of disease and the promotion of optimal health using natural, nontoxic therapies, including diet. In 1940, Henry's son, Victor Lindlahr, MD, followed in his father's footsteps by publishing his groundbreaking book *You Are What You Eat*. He's right.

If you think about it, food is our direct connection to nature. It interacts with our bodies in complex and seemingly magical ways. It plays a major role in the composition of the cells throughout our bodies and influences how we function, think, and even feel. That is pretty magical, right?

Your Body Is Younger Than You Think

You may have heard or read that we replace every cell in our body every seven to ten years. That statement is true with a few exceptions, such as brain cells, so most of our body is under constant renewal and repair. Where does the body get the raw materials for this effort? From food. Scientists are discovering just how effective—seemingly magical—food is in making all of this happen. A healthful diet is one of the reasons we often act and feel younger than our numerical age would indicate.

If we are constantly making new cells and repairing or remodeling others, why do we age? It has to do with several factors but is largely related to a built-in biological clock that is triggered every time a cell replicates itself. As we age, the cumulative effects of cellular and DNA damage make it more difficult for a cell to repair and/or remodel itself. Fortunately, there are a lot of components in food that can slow down the process and perhaps even act as sort of a magic fountain of youth. It helps to have an understanding of how our genes work to see the effect of food on our bodies in general and on our health.

Genetics, Epigenetics, and Nutrition

The Human Genome Project (HGP), an international research project, described, or sequenced, the chemical base pairs that make up the genetic code—the DNA—found in a body's 23 pairs of chromosomes. The "genome" of any individual (except for identical twins) is unique. HGP has provided information about how genes work together, as well as the genetic causes of some diseases. Yet, along the way, scientists realized that genetics alone do not entirely determine our health status. Other factors, including primarily the food we eat, influence the expression of genes and whether we develop certain illnesses.

Our DNA Is Not Necessarily Our Destiny

Our genes need specific instructions on what to do, how to do it, and when. It's amazing that a human liver cell contains the same DNA as a brain cell, yet somehow it knows to replicate itself into a liver cell. If these instructions are not found in our DNA, where do they come from? Scientists have discovered an array of chemical markers and switches along the length of the double helix of DNA. Collectively these factors are referred to as the "epigenome." Think of the DNA as a computer while the epigenome is the software. The hardware is important. The software is what actually tells the DNA what to do.

It was originally thought that an individual's DNA and epigenome were firmly established during early fetal development. We now know that the epigenome can change in response to diet, environmental factors, lifestyle choices, and even the way we think. Damage to the epigenome can produce epimutations. But unlike damage to mutated or defective DNA, epimutations are reversible by various compounds found in food.

Food affects how genes are repaired and remodeled throughout your life. Certainly, there are other factors, such as environmental toxins, stress, and even habitual thoughts and attitude. But the answer lies in understanding how to avoid and/or combat harmful factors while making greater use of the beneficial compounds found in food.

Good Nutrition Lowers the Risk of Genetic Disease Expression

In 2000, a landmark study done at Duke University explored the impact of nutrition and epigenetics. The researchers started with pairs of fat mice with yellow fur that carried the agouti gene, which made them fat and yellow and also dramatically increased their risk of developing cancer and diabetes. The goal was to see if that unfortunate genetic legacy could be changed.

Before the mice were conceived, a test group of mother mice was fed a diet rich in compounds collectively called methyl donors, which included vitamin B_{12}, folic acid, and S-adenosylmethionine (SAMe).

The baby mice were born brown and slender and, as they matured, did not succumb to cancer and diabetes. The nutritional intervention had completely erased the cancerous, diabetic genetic destiny of the agouti mice. Although the brown mice had the same genome as the yellow mice, the expression of the genome was significantly different because of nutritional factors. This is another instance of the magic of food and proof that genetic tendencies can be changed with dietary and nutritional approaches.

Human Twin Studies

Some of the best demonstrations of how diet, lifestyle, and the environment affect genetic expression are based upon studies in identical twins, which result from a fertilized egg splitting into two identical embryos. At birth, their genome is identical, but as the twins age, the genomes change dramatically. By the time the twins are in their fifties, they may have only 3% of their genome in common. In other words, the identical twins are now only 3% identical in regards to their expression of DNA. Food and lifestyle are primarily responsible for these changes.

Personality, values, and behavior are more hardwired than once thought, whereas health and the risk of developing certain diseases are hugely variable. This is important to remember, because it shows that we have some control over our genetic destiny by enlisting the aid of healthful food and good nutrition.

The Pima Indians

The Pima Indian population further illustrates the importance of how diet can affect the body. The Pima Indians of Arizona historically have the highest risk of type 2 diabetes and obesity of any Pima population in the world. Research shows that this is related to diet and lifestyle rather than genetic wiring. The Pimas of Mexico cultivate corn, beans, and potatoes as their main staples, plus a limited amount of seasonal vegetables and fruits such as zucchini, tomatoes, garlic, green peppers, peaches, and apples. The Pimas of Mexico also make heavy use of wild and medicinal plants in their diet and exercise much more. Because they have no electricity or running water in their homes, they have to walk long distances to bring in drinking water or wash their clothes. They use no modern household devices, so food preparation is as close to farm to table as you can get.

In contrast, the Pima Indians of Arizona are largely sedentary and follow the dietary practices of many other Americans. As a result, while roughly 22% of Arizona Pimas have type 2 diabetes and 70% are obese, type 2 diabetes is a rarity in the Mexican Pimas and only about 10% could be classified as obese. The average difference in body weight between the Arizona and Mexican Pimas is more than 60 pounds.

Other racial and ethnic groups besides Pima Indians that have a higher tendency for type 2 diabetes include other Native Americans, African Americans, Hispanic Americans, Asian Americans, Australian Aborigines, and Pacific Islanders. In all of these higher risk groups it's important to note that when they follow the traditional dietary and lifestyle practices of their original culture, the rate of diabetes and obesity is low. The diabetes and other health issues appear when people adopt the typical American high-carb, high-sugar diet and sedentary lifestyle.

Diet Affects Epigenetic Factors in the Development of Alzheimer's Disease

Western dietary patterns—eating lots of sugar, carbohydrates, and the wrong type of fats—contribute to the development of chronic degenerative diseases. Let's take a look at just one disease—Alzheimer's. Many people have had someone close to them develop this degenerative brain disorder with its progressive deterioration of memory and cognition. In the United States, it is now estimated to affect about 20% of individuals between 75 and 84 and 42% of people older than age 85. These numbers are striking when compared to data from the 1960s, when the incidence was only 2% in people over the age of 85. The tremendous increase in AD in people over 85 years of age is often referred to as the "Alzheimer's epidemic."

There are actually two types of Alzheimer's—early onset (EOAD) and late onset (LOAD). EOAD occurs in people 30 to 60 years of age. It is rare, as it represents less than 5% of all people who have AD, and it has a strong genetic component. Most Alzheimer's cases are the late onset form, which develops after 60 years of age. LOAD also has a strong genetic link, but dietary, environmental, and lifestyle factors greatly influence a person's risk of developing the disease.

The primary brain lesions of Alzheimer's disease are the result of deposits of a substance known as beta-amyloid. Although the immune cells in the brain normally remove beta-amyloid and plaque, research has shown that susceptible individuals have a chronic and excessive inflammatory reaction to amyloid proteins in the brain, which can promote Alzheimer's disease.

The tremendous increase in late onset Alzheimer's parallels the rise in type 2 diabetes, a condition that is primarily the result of dietary and lifestyle factors. Specifically, too much sugar, too much of the unhealthy fats, and not enough of the good fats lead to a dampening of the effects of the hormone insulin. When cells throughout the body become resistant to insulin, glucose (blood sugar) cannot enter the cells. As a result, it can oxidize and damage external cell structures, or it can also act like superglue in attaching to receptor sites on cells that monitor body function, much as a thermostat monitors and controls room temperature. If your temperature gauge was stuck at 60°F and the heat was set at 70°F, the thermostat would keep the furnace running no matter how hot it got because the temperature gauge would be telling it that it is only 60°F. When blood sugar levels are too high, they block vital feedback to cells about what is going on, which leads to disruption of proper cellular and body function. That explains why poorly controlled diabetes has so many serious consequences.

Since late onset Alzheimer's is so closely linked to insulin resistance, some researchers have referred to it as diabetes of the brain and even "type 3 diabetes." Individuals with type 2 diabetes have a 1.5- to 4-fold risk of developing LOAD as well as dementia caused by damage to the blood vessels of the brain. Insulin resistance in the brain is associated with poor uptake of glucose by brain cells, causing oxidative damage and localized inflammation that lead to beta-amyloid formation. Hence measures to improve blood sugar control and improve insulin sensitivity appear to be important steps in the prevention of LOAD.

- In regard to the genetics of late onset Alzheimer's, the breakdown of the process to clear beta-amyloid from the brain first involves amyloid binding to apolipoprotein E (ApoE); if beta-amyloid is unbound to ApoE, or "free," it begins to build up and form toxic clusters. There are three forms of ApoE coded for by the APOE gene:

- ApoE2, which is associated with decreased risk of developing LOAD.

- ApoE3, which is the most common form and is not known to affect LOAD risk.

- ApoE4, which is associated with an up to twelve times increased risk of developing LOAD.

So a person's risk of developing late onset Alzheimer's for many years is likely the result of his or her genetic expression of ApoE. People who had ApoE4 were at risk; others were not. But with the huge increase in LOAD development, it is clear that other factors are now the biggest contributors in determining the clearance of beta-amyloid from the brain.

The results of a recent study indicate that diet can influence clearing beta-amyloid. The study involved twenty-seven cognitively normal participants and twenty with mild cognitive impairment suggestive of late onset Alzheimer's. The participants were randomly assigned to one of two diets that were identical in total calories:

- High-fat, high-carbohydrate diet: This diet provided 45% energy from total fat (25% from saturated fat), 35% to 40% from carbohydrates, and 15% to 20% from protein. A typical meal for these participants might have included cheeseburgers, soda, and fries. The diet also had a high glycemic index, meaning that it contained a lot of foods that quickly raised blood sugar levels, such as soft drinks, breads, cereals, and pasta.

- Low-fat, low-glycemic diet: Participants in this group ate food with a low glycemic index and low in fat. This diet consisted of 25% energy from fat (less than 7% from saturated fat), 55% to 60% from carbohydrates, and 15% to 20% from protein. A typical meal in this group was fish, brown rice, and steamed vegetables.

At baseline, the researchers found that those with mild cognitive impairment had a greater fraction of their beta-amyloid in the free state than did the participants with normal mental function. Those carrying the genetic risk factor ApoE4 had an even higher level of free beta-amyloid.

At the end of the study, in people with ApoE2 and ApoE3, the high-fat, high-glycemic diet further increased free beta-amyloid levels, while the low-fat, low-glycemic diet produced significant decreases in free beta-amyloid levels. But the different diets had little impact on free beta-amyloid in individuals with ApoE4.

The study also showed that lower insulin levels were associated with higher levels of free beta-amyloid. Insulin is critical for proper brain function for many reasons. When insulin resistance occurs, as in obesity and type 2 diabetes, higher levels of insulin in the blood result in impaired transport of insulin into the brain. Therefore, low levels of insulin in the cerebrospinal fluid reflect systemic insulin resistance.

In the normal brain, insulin plays an important role in maintaining synapses and memory. So with the lower brain insulin levels noted in this study and others, it seems appropriate that LOAD is often referred to as "type 3 diabetes."

These results mean that in individuals who have a low risk of developing late onset Alzheimer's because of their ApoE type, a high-fat, high-glycemic diet produces the same sort of changes in beta-amyloid seen in those with the ApoE4 genetic predisposition to LOAD. In other words, dietary habits can nullify the protection that a person's genetic code can provide. On the flip side, the dietary changes used in this study were not enough to reduce the genetic predisposition toward LOAD in high-risk subjects. Yet that does not mean the disease is inevitable, just that additional dietary and supplement strategies are necessary to address this predisposition.

How Food Interacts with Our Genes

New research reveals ways in which foods seem to interact magically with our genes and epigenetics.

One discovery is that plant foods contain small fragments of RNA (ribonucleic acid), which are now known to modify genetic behavior. One form of RNA is called messenger RNA, or mRNA (which is basically more "software"), because it instructs various cells to assemble a specific protein or perform some other vital task. Another type of RNA found in plants is composed of small fragments called microRNAs (miRNAs), which play a huge role in how cells grow and die and how cell functions are balanced in their input and output of energy.

Chinese scientists used Japanese honeysuckle (*Lonicera japonica*), a remedy for colds and influenza in traditional Chinese medicine, to show how its miRNA can help in viral infections. The study showed that, when mice drank honeysuckle tea, the miRNA traveled via the bloodstream to the lungs, where it directly targeted the influenza A virus. This group of viruses is the culprit behind the Spanish flu, swine flu, and avian flu epidemics. So here we have an herb with a historical use for symptoms related to what we now know are caused by viruses, showing significant activity against these viruses in a newly discovered mechanism. Before this model existed, all that was known was that the herb exerted some sort of magical effect against viral infections.

Additional studies have shown that concentrated plant miRNAs are successful in reducing the number of tumors in animals with colon cancer.

We Are Biochemically Unique

In the late 1970s, when I began discovering the importance of nutrition in human health, one of my heroes was Roger Williams, who was responsible for discovering many B vitamins, including pantothenic acid and folic acid.

One of the most important concepts that Dr. Williams introduced was the idea of "biochemical individuality." Each of us has unique biochemical traits that determine who we are and how we interact with the world around us. Biochemical individuality is what makes all of us unique in the interaction between our genes and our environment. It also plays a big role in determining how healthy we are and what ailments we are likely to experience.

What determines our biochemical individuality is a family of perhaps one hundred enzymes within our cells known as the cytochrome P450 enzymes. These enzymes play a critical role in processing food components as well as detoxifying drugs, cancer-causing compounds, and hormones. Generally, each enzyme is designed to metabolize certain types of chemicals, but there is also a lot of functional overlap. This "backup system" ensures that your liver is usually able to detoxify your body efficiently.

Nutrigenomics may clarify the effects of dietary practices. Differences in these enzymes may explain why some people can smoke without developing lung cancer and why certain individuals are more susceptible to the harmful effects of pesticides and other toxic chemicals.

Research on the effects of coffee consumption on heart disease has been a mixed bag: one study finds no correlation between coffee consumption and heart disease, while another shows a correlation with heart attack risk, yet another shows elevated cholesterol for those drinking more than four cups, and still another shows no correlation when paper filters are used.

Let's take a look at a study examining the association between heart attack rates and caffeine consumption. Unlike other studies, this one also measured the activity of the liver enzyme that detoxifies caffeine. Researchers divided the group according to whether they possessed a form of this enzyme that metabolized caffeine quickly or slowly. Those with the rapid caffeine breakdown decreased their risk of a heart attack by drinking coffee, while slow caffeine metabolizers dramatically increased their risk. Drinking four cups a day of coffee was associated with a 17% decreased risk in fast metabolizers and a 260% increased risk in slow metabolizers.

Many drugs, hormones, and dietary factors also influence this enzyme system. For example, the enzyme system is inhibited by oral contraceptives and enhanced by vegetables in the cabbage family. In addition, there is convincing evidence that regular coffee consumption decreases the risk of developing Parkinson's disease, Alzheimer's disease, and type 2 diabetes.

In the future, nutrigenomics will enable us to use food prescriptions to influence gene expression so as to promote health based upon our individual biochemical makeup. Many mechanisms of health-promoting components of food are now being uncovered. I will explain how you can take advantage of this new knowledge so that the food you eat will dramatically improve your health. It is an exciting dawn of an emerging era with so much that can be applied today to start helping you.

What Should We Eat for Health and Longevity?

To identify the best foods to eat for health and longevity, it makes sense to look at the lifestyles of people who enjoy good health, vitality, and longevity. A few dietary patterns that are associated with health and longevity stand out, such as the Mediterranean diet, the Okinawan diet, and the New Nordic diet.

My goal is to show you that these diets are similar in their food groups even though they differ significantly in the actual foods. I've used the best practices from all of these diets, as well as the latest scientific information on nutrition, to weave together my Synergetic Diet. The Synergetic Diet brings together healing forces that certain foods and their components exert on our health and well-being to provide a healthy eating and weight-loss program.

In the Beginning

Humans evolved with the capacity to digest meat and other animal proteins, such as dairy products, and plant foods. But several physical characteristics in our gastrointestinal tract indicate that we are best designed to eat plant foods. Whereas most carnivores have a short intestinal tract, the human gastrointestinal tract is 30 feet long. Most carnivorous animals have a mouthful of sharp canine teeth, whereas only our front four canine teeth are designed for meat eating. The rest are perfect for biting, crushing, and grinding plant foods. So as far as our eating machinery goes, it looks as though we are designed primarily, but not exclusively, to be vegetarians.

The diet of wild primates—chimpanzees, monkeys, and gorillas—gives us clues as to what we should eat. Research has shown that only about 2% of our calories should come from meat, based upon our smaller size relative to gorillas and orangutans. Those primates are what we call opportunistic carnivores. They eat mainly fruits and vegetables but, if the opportunity arises, may also eat small animals, lizards, and eggs. Unfortunately, the cultivated fruits in American supermarkets is much less nutritious than the wild fruits those animals rely on, so we need to make some dietary adjustments.

The biggest difference between humans and apes is that our brains are bigger and metabolically more active. The prehistoric shift to animal foods may have been the stimulus for the growth of the human brain. With a bigger brain, early humans could engage in more complex social behavior, leading to improved foraging and hunting tactics, which in turn led to even higher quality food intake, fostering brain evolution and on and on.

What We Eat Today

During the twentieth century, our food consumption patterns changed for the worse, after thousands of years of hunting, gathering, and agriculture. Based on USDA data, total dietary fat intake rose from 32% of calories in 1909 to 43% by 2000. Overall carbohydrate intake dropped from 57% to 46%, while protein intake has remained at about 11%. These detrimental dietary changes have come from unwise individual food choices as society has shifted away from whole, unprocessed foods to processed foods containing too much salt, sugar, and artificial ingredients such as trans fatty acids. Currently, more than half of the carbohydrates being consumed in the United States are in the form of sugars, such as sucrose and high-fructose corn syrup, which are added to processed foods as sweetening agents.

Looking at Healthful Diets Around the Globe

It is now well established that certain dietary practices can cause—and others can prevent—a wide range of diseases, particularly chronic degenerative diseases such as heart disease, cancer, and other conditions associated with aging. Recent research indicates that certain diets and foods provide immediate therapeutic benefit as well. It's been proved that (1) a diet rich in plant foods (whole grains, legumes, nuts and seeds, fruits, and vegetables) is protective against many diseases that are common in Western society and (2) a diet that has a low percentage of plant foods is a causative factor in the development of these diseases and creates conditions under which other causative factors are more active.

Much of the link between diet and chronic disease originated from the work of two medical pioneers, Denis Burkitt, MD, and Hubert Trowell, MD, the authors of *Western Diseases: Their Emergence and Prevention*. Based on extensive studies examining the rates of diseases in various populations (epidemiologic data) and his own observations of primitive cultures, Burkitt established four stages in the development of Western diseases:

- First stage: In cultures consuming a traditional diet consisting of whole, unprocessed foods, the rate of chronic diseases such as heart disease, diabetes, and cancer is quite low.

- Second stage: As people begin to eat a more "Western" diet, there is a sharp rise in the number of individuals with obesity and diabetes.

- Third stage: As more people abandon their traditional diet, conditions that were once quite rare become common, such as constipation, hemorrhoids, varicose veins, and appendicitis.

- Fourth stage: With full Westernization of the diet, other chronic degenerative or potentially lethal diseases become common, such as heart disease, cancer, osteoarthritis, rheumatoid arthritis, and gout.

Since Burkitt and Trowell's pioneering research, a virtual landslide of data has continually verified the role of diet as the key factor in almost every chronic disease, especially obesity and diabetes.

The truth is that virtually any traditional diet from anywhere on the globe is bound to provide more health benefits than the standard American diet, because traditional diets focus on whole, natural, unprocessed foods.

The Seven Countries Study

One of the most important scientific studies to look at the role of diet began in 1956 under the direction of Ancel Keys, PhD, from the University of Minnesota. The study sought to examine the relationships among lifestyle and diet, coronary heart disease, and stroke in various populations around the world. Like all studies, it had its limitations, but it was truly a game changer and continues to provide valuable data to this day.

Initially, the Seven Countries Study enrolled 12,763 men, 40 to 59 years of age, from seven countries in four regions (United States, northern Europe, southern Europe, and Japan). The subjects were separated into sixteen groups: one in the United States; two in Finland; one in the Netherlands; three in Italy; five in Yugoslavia (two in Croatia and three in Serbia); two in Greece; and two in Japan.

One of the main findings of the study was that diet and lifestyle definitely affected the risk and rates of heart attacks and strokes. Deaths from cardiovascular disease in the United States and northern Europe greatly exceeded those in southern Europe, even when controlled for factors such as age, cholesterol, blood pressure, smoking, physical activity, and weight. In other words, diet was critical in causing or preventing heart disease. The Seven Countries Study also supported what Burkitt and Trowell observed: When people changed their diet habits from their traditional one to a more Westernized one, there was a significant increase in the risk of heart disease. Three diets that are associated with a lower risk of heart disease are described next.

The Mediterranean Diet

The Mediterranean diet refers to eating patterns typical of southern European regions, such as Crete, parts of Greece, and southern Italy. It includes several characteristic foods and dietary practices:

- Extra-virgin olive oil is the principal source of fat for cooking and eating. Eating an abundance of seasonally fresh and locally grown foods, including fruits, vegetables, beans, nuts, and seeds.

- Foods are minimally processed.

- Fresh fruits are eaten for dessert, with sweets containing concentrated sugars or honey consumed a few times per week at the most.

- Dairy products, principally cheese and yogurt, are consumed daily in low to moderate amounts.

- Seafood is eaten frequently; red meat and poultry less so.

- Poultry and eggs are consumed in moderate amounts (one to four times weekly) or not at all.

- Pasta, bread, and grains are consumed in moderation.

- Wine is consumed in low to moderate amounts with meals.

For many reasons, olive oil gets a lot of credit for the health benefits of the traditional Mediterranean diet. But the research clearly shows that there is a significant synergy among all the components of the diet rather than one specific factor responsible for all the benefits.

The Okinawan Diet

Okinawa is the largest of the Ryukyu Islands of Japan. Its inhabitants, who have a life expectancy among the highest in the world, are known for their low rate of obesity and low mortality rate from cardiovascular disease and many types of cancer. In this study, when compared to Americans, an average Okinawan was 8 times less likely to die from coronary heart disease, 7 times less likely to die from prostate cancer, 6.5 times less likely to die from breast cancer, and 2.5 times less likely to die from colon cancer than an average American of the same age.

Okinawans consume only 30% of the rice and other foods from grains common to the Japanese diet. Instead, the purple-fleshed Okinawan sweet potato is the main source of complex carbohydrates. In the 1950s, the sweet potato contributed nearly 70% of the total calories consumed by the Okinawans.

For the most part, the daily diet was almost entirely plant based. Most meals featured sweet potato, leafy green or yellow root vegetables, and soy products (e.g., miso soup, tofu, edamame). Smaller servings of fish, noodles, or lean meats flavored with herbs and spices often accompanied those main staples. Pork was eaten primarily on special occasions.

The Okinawan diet was created out of necessity. In the first half of the twentieth century, meat was too expensive for the average Asian family. The same was true of many processed foods, including polished white rice, sugar, salt, and cooking oil. Climate also played a role, as Okinawa is a subtropical island with seasonal, quite severe storms. The sweet potato is so hardy that it can survive severe tropical storms, and it has two growing seasons. Okinawans ate what they could grow, catch, and harvest.

The traditional dietary pattern in Okinawa has the following characteristics, typical of other healthful diets:

- Low caloric intake
- Low fat intake, with a high ratio of mono- and polyunsaturated fats to saturated fats, and a low omega 6:3 ratio (discussed in chapter 4)
- High consumption of vegetables, particularly sweet potatoes and other root and green-yellow vegetables

- High consumption of legumes, mostly soybeans
- Moderate consumption of fish products, with higher consumption along coastal areas
- Low consumption of meat and dairy products
- Moderate alcohol consumption

That was the traditional Okinawan diet until the 1960s, when people began eating a more Western and Japanese diet. Fat intake rose from 10% to 27% of total calorie intake, and the sweet potato was replaced by rice and bread. Not surprisingly, the health patterns of Okinawans are being adversely affected by these changes.

Rarely does one vegetable constitute such a major caloric content of a population's diet. Since the sweet potato accounted for such a large percentage of calories (roughly 70%) of the Okinawan diet, a strong case could be made that that vegetable was the key factor in the good health that population enjoyed. Of course, it was the synergetic effects of their entire diet that rounded out the dietary benefits.

The sweet potato is a member of the morning glory (*Convolvulaceae*) family. It is native to Central America and has been consumed since prehistoric times, making it one of the oldest known vegetables. Christopher Columbus was the first explorer to take the sweet potato back to Europe. Later Spanish and Portuguese explorers further spread the sweet potato by carrying it to Africa, India, Indonesia, and southern Asia. The sweet potato was taken to the Okinawan Islands by Chinese traders in the 1600s.

Sweet potatoes in Okinawa come in purple, violet, yellow, red, and orange shades. In the United States, the orange-fleshed sweet potato is often referred to as a yam to distinguish it from the white-fleshed Irish potato. But technically it is not a yam, as true yams are native to Africa and are distinct in flavor. Sweet potatoes are an excellent source of carotenes—the darker the variety, the higher the concentration of carotenes—and can be roasted, baked, or mashed. They are also a good source of vitamins C, B_2, and B_6, manganese, copper, biotin, pantothenic acid, and dietary fiber.

The special health benefits of sweet potatoes may come from their unique root storage proteins, which are shown to exert significant antioxidant effects.

One of the biggest health benefits of sweet potatoes is that, unlike many other starchy root vegetables, they are considered an "antidiabetic" food, as they help stabilize blood sugar levels. In fact, sweet potatoes have been promoted in traditional Japanese medicine as a remedy for diabetes, and extracts of the white-skinned variety are approved in Japan as a functional food in the treatment of type 2 diabetes. This extract lowers blood glucose by increasing insulin sensitivity. This effect is important not only in lowering blood sugar levels but also in fighting against obesity and heart disease. Sweet potatoes exert some interesting antiobesity effects, indicating that they might have been one of the key reasons the Okinawans enjoyed such good health over all those many years. Of course, there are other medicinal foods in the Okinawan diet that you will learn about in subsequent chapters, including turmeric, seaweed, and mushrooms.

The New Nordic Diet

In the Seven Countries Study, the traditional Nordic dietary pattern was associated with greater heart disease risk in Norway, Sweden, Denmark, Finland, and Iceland. Those countries took this information and acted on it by creating a New Nordic diet with the help of researchers, nutritionists, and chefs at the University of Copenhagen in 2004. Their goal was to define a new regional cuisine to combat growing rates of not only heart disease but also obesity, diabetes, and cancer.

Like the Mediterranean diet, the New Nordic diet focuses on eating whole foods and plant foods that are indigenous to Nordic countries. The diet includes:

- Eat more plants, including root and cruciferous vegetables, dark leafy greens, apples and pears, and berries (e.g., lingonberries and bilberries).
- Eat more whole grains, especially rye and oats.
- Eat more high protein, omega-3-rich fish and shellfish from cold waters that have low mercury levels.
- Eat smaller portions of meat and dairy products, choosing lean meats such as venison and elk over beef.

- Include locally foraged foods such as moss, mushrooms, nettles, sea vegetables, garlic, and even ants.
- Use fresh herbs, including dill, chives, and fennel, abundantly.

Several studies have validated the diet's health benefits, including an ability to lower cholesterol and blood pressure, reduce systemic inflammation, and help people lose weight. In a study conducted in Denmark, overweight subjects followed either the New Nordic diet or the "traditional Danish diet." Food was supplied free of charge and intake was monitored, but test subjects were allowed to eat as much as they wanted and could occasionally deviate from the prescribed plan. After six months, those who followed the New Nordic diet had consumed fewer calories each day over a six-month period. The average weight loss was about 10 pounds for the New Nordic participants compared to 3 pounds for the traditional Danish diet group. The New Nordic diet also produced greater reductions in systolic blood pressure and diastolic blood pressure than did the typical Danish diet.

In another study led by the Institute of Public Health and Clinical Nutrition at the University of Eastern Finland, the New Nordic diet demonstrated an ability to reduce the expression of inflammation-associated genes in fat cells in obese subjects with the metabolic syndrome. Results showed differences in the function of as many as 128 different genes in the fat cells of the New Nordic diet group compared with the control group. If you can influence genes in this manner, you are helping your cells work more efficiently at reducing obesity and inflammation.

The Synergetic Diet

I have created the Synergetic Diet, which incorporates the best of the most healthful diets highlighted in this chapter and more.

People who include a variety of different foods in their diets have a lower rate of obesity than those who consume the same foods day in and day out. Most Americans eat a limited, monotonous range of foods. It is entirely possible that excessive calorie and food consumption may be some sort of physiological craving gone awry. In other words, the brain might be seeking to improve the body's nutritional intake by sending signals to eat, but the signals are nonspecific and simply result in eating more calories not necessarily the specific nutrients the brain needs to feel satisfied.

A study by researchers at the Harvard School of Public Health and the New York University School of Medicine provides some evidence that dietary variety may help prevent obesity. To evaluate the role of food variety on body weight, researchers evaluated dietary data from the National Health and Nutrition Examination Survey (NHANES), conducted from 2003 to 2006, of more than seven thousand men and nonpregnant, nonlactating women aged 20 and older. The subjects were divided into groups 1 through 5, with the higher number reflecting greater dietary variety. Both the men and women in the group with the greatest degree of dietary variety had a roughly 50% reduced risk of being obese. Those results indicate that greater dietary variety is inversely associated with obesity in both sexes. Eating a variety of nutritious foods may protect against excess body weight. This study explicitly recognizes the potential benefits of dietary variety in obesity management and provides the foundation to support its ongoing evaluation.

Consuming a broad range of food components plays an important role in promoting human health. We need variety in our diet to make sure we are getting the full spectrum of protection. A varied diet makes our food choices more interesting and less boring. Eating the same foods again and again is a sure path to food boredom. Dietary variety wakes up the senses and makes eating more interesting and fun.

One of my goals in writing this book is to instill the importance of eating a wider spectrum of health-promoting foods. *The Magic of Food* is meant to help you appreciate how eating a wide variety of foods can improve your health and well-being. Open your eyes and mouth, and take advantage of the incredible bounty of foods that is available to you!

AMPk: Activating the Enzyme of Youth, Longevity, and Weight Loss

AMP-activated protein kinase, or AMPk, is an enzyme produced by the body that has the magical ability to burn fat and turn up your metabolism. AMPk is found in every cell and serves as a master regulating switch in energy metabolism. This enzyme plays a major role in determining body fat composition, especially the amount of visceral belly fat that we carry. Its activity is also tied to our life expectancy. When we are young, AMPk is more active, but as we age, cellular AMPk activation decreases, leading to belly (visceral) fat accumulation and loss of muscle mass. Low AMPk activity is also linked to chronic inflammation, high blood cholesterol and triglyceride levels, insulin resistance, mitochondrial insufficiency and dysfunction, brain cell degeneration, obesity, and poor blood sugar control.

The good news is that researchers are discovering natural and positive ways to enhance AMPk with specific dietary strategies and food components. Not surprisingly, these natural approaches hold great promise in the goal of near-effortless weight loss as a result. The most important influencer of AMPk activity appears to be the sensitivity of cells to the hormone insulin. As a result, with insulin resistance there is reduced AMPk activity.

Insulin resistance is closely tied to abdominal obesity and type 2 diabetes. If your waist circumference is larger than hip circumference, there is a likelihood that you suffer from insulin resistance. As the number and size of fat cells increase, they lead to a reduction in the secretion of compounds that promote insulin action, including a protein produced by fat cells known as adiponectin. Making matters worse is the fact that there is also an increase in the secretion of a substance called resistin, which dampens the effect of insulin.

Adiponectin increases the activation of AMPk, while resistin impairs AMPk activity. So whereas adiponectin is associated with improved insulin sensitivity and metabolism, resistin is associated with poor blood sugar control, increased blood lipid levels, and the development of atherosclerosis. All of these effects are due to the influence these compounds have on AMPk activity.

The first step in improving AMPk activity is to improve insulin sensitivity. By doing so, adiponectin levels are increased and resistin levels are lowered, which in turn leads to AMPk activation.

How Do You Know If You Are Insulin Resistant?

One of the most useful clinical determinants of insulin resistance is to measure the waist-to-hip ratio. If a man's waist circumference is greater than 40 inches or a woman's is greater than 35 inches, there is no need to do any further calculation, because this measurement alone has been shown to be a major risk factor in both heart disease and type 2 diabetes, two of the biggest consequences of insulin resistance. A waist-to-hip ratio greater than 1.0 for men and 0.8 for women is highly predictive of insulin resistance. To determine your waist-to-hip ratio:

1. Measure the circumference of your waist: _____
2. Measure the circumference of your hips: _____
3. Divide the waist measurement by the hip measurement:
   Waist/hip _____. This is your waist-to-hip ratio.

Insulin Resistance and Cardiovascular Disease

Insulin resistance occurs when your body becomes less sensitive to the actions of your own insulin. One of the key actions of insulin is to drive glucose from the blood into the cells. Insulin resistance leads to elevations in blood sugar levels and is tied closely to obesity and type 2 diabetes. Insulin resistance is also linked to an increased risk of developing heart disease, certain cancers, and Alzheimer's disease (see page 5). Let's take a look at how insulin resistance impacts heart disease.

- Elevated blood sugar levels are associated with increased attachment of glucose to receptor proteins, leading to loss of key feedback mechanisms. For example, if the receptor for low-density lipoprotein cholesterol (LDL; "bad" cholesterol) on the surface of a liver cell becomes damaged by the attachment of glucose, the liver cell does not receive the feedback message that there is plenty of circulating cholesterol. In the absence of feedback, the liver cell thinks it needs to make more cholesterol.

- Elevated levels of blood sugar are also associated with increased oxidative stress and damage to LDL cholesterol. This adds fuel to the fire of silent inflammation. In fact, insulin resistance is the key factor in causing silent inflammation and high levels of high-sensitivity C-reactive protein (hsCRP), a blood marker of inflammation. Much of the inflammatory effect of insulin resistance is due to its negative effects on the endothelium, the lining of the blood vessel wall.

- Since there is a relative deficiency of glucose within cells because of insulin resistance, even though blood sugar levels are high, the pancreas begins dumping larger quantities of insulin into the blood. High blood insulin levels are now a well-established risk factor for heart disease. A high level of insulin in the blood promotes atherosclerosis by several mechanisms, including stimulating smooth muscle cell proliferation in the arterial wall, leading to thickening and stiffness of the arterial wall and narrowing of the artery.

• Insulin resistance is also associated with high blood pressure. Insulin resistance not only contributes to blood vessels becoming more rigid and constricted but also causes retention of sodium and water from the kidneys, which results in high blood pressure.

• Insulin resistance promotes greater fat breakdown, leading to the characteristic blood lipid pattern of elevated LDL and triglyceride levels with lower levels of high-density-lipoprotein cholesterol (HDL, or "good" cholesterol). In healthy individuals, one of the functions of insulin is to suppress the breakdown of fat from the fat cells into the bloodstream. With insulin resistance this effect is blocked, leading to an exaggerated breakdown of fat from the fat cells and the release of free fatty acids into the blood. The liver takes up these free fatty acids and converts them into triglycerides in the form of very-low-density lipoprotein (VLDL), which ultimately lowers HDL levels. Insulin resistance also increases the formation of the smaller, denser LDL, which is damaging to arteries.

• Insulin resistance greatly increases the risk of blood clot formation and blocks the action of tissue plasminogen activator, a clot-busting compound produced by the cells that line the arteries.

• Insulin resistance is associated with increased levels of the adrenal hormone cortisol.

When it comes to insulin resistance, here are some sobering facts. It is currently estimated that eight out of ten adults in the United States are overweight. About half of these people, 40% of our adult population, meet the criteria of being obese. Obese individuals have an average life expectancy five to seven years shorter than that of normal-weight individuals. Most of the increased risk of mortality is due to heart disease, because obesity carries with it a significant risk of type 2 diabetes, elevated cholesterol levels, high blood pressure, and other risk factors for the development of atherosclerosis (hardening of the arteries). Increased medical expenses due to the overweight and obese population in the United States are estimated at more than $200 billion per year.

In addition to the obesity epidemic, there is a parallel epidemic of type 2 diabetes. Currently, twenty million Americans meet the criteria for type 2 diabetes and another eighty million suffer from prediabetes—a condition characterized by insulin resistance—and/or metabolic syndrome. All told, more than one hundred million people in the United States show signs of significant insulin resistance.

A combination of the lifestyle changes described in the Synergetic Diet—increasing physical activity, improving diet and nutrition, and using targeted nutritional supplementation—will help you lose weight and improve your insulin sensitivity.

How to Improve Insulin Sensitivity by Using the Glycemic Index

Dietary carbohydrates play a central role in the cause, prevention, and treatment of insulin resistance and type 2 diabetes. In the effort to label carbohydrate sources as good or bad, one useful tool is the glycemic index (GI). It is a numerical scale used to indicate how fast and how high a particular food raises blood glucose levels compared with glucose. Refined sugars, white flour products, and other sources of simple sugars are quickly absorbed into the bloodstream, causing a rapid rise in blood sugar levels, severely stressing blood sugar control and insulin resistance. This effect is why it's important to avoid eating processed foods and certain fruits and vegetables.

Studies have shown that an elevated after-meal blood sugar level is a greater risk factor for heart disease than an abnormal fasting plasma glucose level. So even if you do not have insulin resistance, it is essential to avoid high blood sugar levels at any time to prevent a potential heart attack or stroke.

Though the GI is quite useful, it doesn't tell you how many carbohydrates are in a serving of a particular food, so another tool is needed. The glycemic load (GL) is a relatively new way to assess the impact of carbohydrate consumption. It takes the glycemic index into account but gives a more complete picture of the effect that a particular food has on blood sugar levels based on how much carbohydrate there is in a serving. A GL of 20 or more is high, a GL of 11 to 19 is medium, and a GL of 10 or less is low.

Let's take a look at beets, which have a high GI but low GL. Although the carbohydrate in beets has a high GI, there isn't a lot of it, so a typical serving of cooked beets has a low GL, about 5. As long as you eat a reasonable portion of a low-glycemic-load food, the impact on blood sugar is acceptable, even if the food has a high GI.

Examples of Glycemic Index, Glycemic Load, and Insulin Stress Scores of Selected Foods			
Food	Glycemic Index	Glycemic Load	Insulin Stress (Glycemic Impact)
Carrots, cooked, ½ cup	49	1.5	Low
Peach, fresh, 1 large	42	3.0	Low
Beets, cooked, ½ cup	64	3.0	Low
Watermelon, ½ cup	72	4.0	Low
Whole wheat bread, 1 slice	69	9.6	Low
Baked potato, medium	93	14	Medium
Brown rice, cooked, 1 cup	50	16	Medium
Banana, raw, 1 medium	55	17.6	Medium
Spaghetti, white, cooked, 1 cup	41	23	High
White rice, cooked, 1 cup	72	26	High
Grape Nuts cereal, ½ cup	71	33	Very high
Soft drinks, 375 ml	68	34.7	Very high

In essence, foods that are mostly water (e.g., apples and watermelon), fiber (e.g., beets and carrots), or air (e.g., popcorn) will not cause a steep rise in your blood sugar even if their GI is high, as long as you exercise moderation in portion sizes. I recommend keeping the GL for any three-hour period to less than 20. The reason is that each time a food containing carbohydrate is eaten, it can produce a further increase in blood sugar levels. Three hours are usually required for blood sugar levels to drop back to those prior to the preceding meal.

To download a full Glycemic Load of Foods Table with over 230 foods listed, go to www.doctormurray.com/glycemic-load.

How Dietary Fiber Improves Insulin Sensitivity

Population studies, as well as clinical and experimental data, show diabetes to be one of the diseases most related to inadequate dietary fiber intake. Different types of fibers possess different actions. The type of fiber that exerts the most beneficial effects on blood sugar control is the water-soluble form. Particularly good food sources of water-soluble fiber are beans, peas, and lentils; most vegetables; nuts; seeds; oat bran; citrus fruits; pears; and apples. These types of fiber-rich foods can help to slow down the digestion and absorption of carbohydrates, thereby preventing rapid rises in blood sugar. Eating legumes, in particular, is associated with increasing the sensitivity of tissues to insulin and improving the uptake of glucose by the muscles, liver, and other tissues, thereby preventing a sustained elevation of blood sugar. My recommendation is to consume at least 35 grams of fiber a day from various food sources, especially vegetables. You can track your fiber intake with the help of apps like My Fit Life and Food Tracker.

For people seeking to improve blood sugar control, I also recommend taking a dietary fiber supplement at all meals. There are several sources that exert significant effects in helping to stabilize blood sugar levels as well as produce a myriad of other health benefits. The best research is on a dietary fiber matrix called PolyGlycopleX (PGX®) as well as psyllium seed husks (e.g., Metamucil), guar gum, pectin, and resistant dextrin (e.g., tapioca fiber). Information on which specific dietary fibers can help reduce blood sugar levels and improve blood sugar control is provided beginning on page 116.

Legumes: An Antidiabetes Food That Activates AMPk

Fossil records show that legumes are among the oldest cultivated plants. Prehistoric people domesticated and cultivated certain legumes for food. Today, legumes are regularly eaten in most diets of the world. There are more than thirteen thousand legume species, second only to grains in supplying calories and protein to the world's population. Compared to grains, legumes supply about the same number of total calories but usually provide two to four times as much protein.

Although legumes are often called "the poor person's meat," a better name would be "the healthy person's meat." Their major health benefit is that they are a rich source of soluble fiber. In addition to lowering cholesterol, the high fiber content of legumes prevents blood sugar levels from rising too rapidly after a meal, making them an especially good choice for individuals with diabetes and/or insulin resistance. They are also activators of AMPk, making them important in any weight-loss plan.

The Importance of Preventing Glycation

One of the theories regarding aging is related to excessive attachment of blood sugar (glucose) molecules to cellular proteins. This process, called glycation or glycosylation, can wreak havoc on cellular function. For example, cholesterol-carrying proteins that have been glycosylated do not bind to receptors on liver cells that halt the manufacture of cholesterol. As a result, there is a loss of natural feedback and the liver thinks it needs to make more cholesterol because it is not getting the signal to stop.

Excessive glycation also leads to the formation of advanced glycation end products (AGEs). AGEs have many adverse effects: they inactivate enzymes, damage structural and regulatory proteins, impair immune function, and increase the likelihood of developing autoimmune diseases. Like free-radical damage, AGEs are associated with many chronic degenerative diseases. Diets that promote glycation and poor glucose control cause decreased AMPk activity, leading to accelerated cellular aging, obesity, and the development of chronic degenerative diseases such as cancers, heart disease, Alzheimer's disease, and macular degeneration.

To avoid excessive glycation, the Synergetic Diet is the key. Blood sugar levels are controlled by consuming a low-glycemic diet and, if needed, using nutritional supplements. Especially helpful are soluble dietary fiber supplements such as PGX, psyllium seed husks (e.g., Metamucil), guar gum, pectin, and resistant dextrin (e.g., tapioca fiber).

The target threshold for blood sugar levels to prevent excessive glycation is less than 140 mg/ml one or two hours after a meal. Diabetics are often told to keep the level below 180 mg/ml, but that is too high for good health and will lead to excessive glycation.

Dietary Fat and Insulin Resistance

Dietary fat also plays a central role in insulin sensitivity. Insulin resistance is linked to eating an abundance of saturated fat from animal foods and trans fatty acids (partially hydrogenated vegetable oils) rather than healthy mono-unsaturated and omega-3 fatty acids. It seems that dietary fat determines cell membrane composition and such a dietary pattern leads to reduced membrane fluidity, which in turn causes reduced insulin binding to receptors on cellular membranes, reduced insulin action, or both.

The key is to rely on monounsaturated fats and omega-3 oils, which improve insulin action as well as AMPk activity. Clinical, as well as population-based studies, indicate that frequent consumption of mono-unsaturated fats such as extra-virgin olive oil, raw or lightly roasted nuts and seeds, nut oils, and omega-3 fatty acids from fish protect against the development of type 2 diabetes. Healthy omega-3 fish include wild salmon, trout, anchovies, sardines, halibut, and herring. The evidence indicates that altered cell membrane composition and fluidity play a critical role in the development of type 2 diabetes.

Studies have shown that consumption of nuts is inversely associated with risk of type 2 diabetes, independent of known risk factors, including age, obesity, family history of diabetes, physical inactivity, smoking, and other dietary factors. In addition to providing beneficial monounsaturated and polyunsaturated fats that improve insulin sensitivity, nuts are rich in fiber and magnesium and have a low GI. Higher intakes of fiber, magnesium, and foods with a low GI have been associated with a reduced risk of developing type 2 diabetes in several population-based studies. Eating mostly raw or lightly roasted fresh nuts and seeds rather than commercially roasted and salted nuts and seeds is advocated. I recommend eating ¼ to ½ cup of nuts daily.

Additional Factors That Activate AMPk

In addition to improving insulin sensitivity and consuming more soluble fiber, there are many other factors that activate AMPk. Several of these are discussed in other chapters, including:

- Intense exercise

- Calorie restriction

- Thyroid hormone

- Adiponectin

- Good oils, including extra-virgin olive oil, avocado oil, macadamia nut oil, fish oils (EPA+DHA), and oils containing medium-chain triglycerides (such as coconut oil)

- Various plant factors (flavonoids, polyphenols, carotenes, etc.): anthocyanins (blueberries and other berries), catechins (green tea), flavonols (cacao, cocoa, and dark chocolate), fucoidan (brown seaweed), genistein (soy), polymethoxylated flavones (citrus fruits), procyanidolic oligomers (grape seeds), and resveratrol (red wine and Chinese knotweed)

- Numerous spices, herbs, and herbal compounds: berberine (goldenseal, coptis, etc.), black pepper, cayenne pepper, cinnamon, garlic, onions, ginger, green coffee bean extract, mint-family herbs (basil, oregano, rosemary, sage, and thyme), mulberry leaf, and turmeric

- Health-promoting probiotics such as *Lactobacillus* species

Remember that inhibitors of AMPk include:

- Insulin resistance
- High-fat diet
- Caloric excess
- Sedentary lifestyle
- Aging

Dietary Supplements and Herbal Products That Activate AMPk

Many dietary supplements and herbal products activate AMPk and may help people lose weight.

In regard to dietary supplements, compounds that enhance the function of the mitochondria, the energy-producing factories in our cells, such as alpha-lipoic acid (ALA), creatine, carnitine, and coenzyme Q10 may be helpful. Of these substances, ALA is the best choice.

ALA is a naturally occurring and necessary biological factor in our cells. Although it has some vitaminlike functions, as it can be synthesized in the body, it is not classified as a vitamin. The medical use of ALA has focused on its positive effects in patients with diabetes. Double-blind clinical trials in humans have demonstrated that it improves insulin sensitivity, blood sugar control, cardiovascular health, nerve function, and lipid levels and reduces symptoms of diabetic neuropathy.

Recent preclinical studies have indicated that ALA may help to boost metabolism, promote the burning of fat as energy, reduce food intake, and therefore potentially aid in weight loss. The same is true of the long-chain omega-3 fatty acid eicosapentaenoic acid (EPA), found in fish oil. When researchers sought to better clarify the weight loss–promoting effects of ALA and EPA, 97 overweight or obese women were put on a weight loss–promoting diet of 30% less than total energy expenditure. The women were then divided into four groups. One group served as the control group; the others were given either ALA, 300 mg; EPA, 1.3 grams; or ALA, 300 mg, and EPA, 1.3 grams.

The study lasted ten weeks. Results showed that ALA supplementation alone or in combination with EPA enhanced the effects of dieting. The control group lost an average of 11.44 pounds; the EPA group, 11.88 pounds; the ALA group, 15.4 pounds; and the ALA + EPA group, 14.3 pounds. Hence, taking 300 mg of ALA brought about approximately 4 pounds of extra weight loss over the course of the ten weeks.

Three herbal products that can activate AMPk stand out:

1. Berberine is a naturally occurring alkaloid found in many medicinal plant species worldwide, including barberry (*Berberis vulgaris*), Chinese goldthread (*Coptis chinensis*), and goldenseal (*Hydrastis canadensis*). They are potent activators of AMPk and have shown impressive results in improving blood sugar control, enhancing insulin sensitivity, and lowering blood pressure in overweight subjects, with modest benefits in weight loss as well. In one double-blind study, subjects taking berberine at a dosage of 500 mg three times daily before meals for three months compared to a placebo group showed a significant decrease in waist circumference (106 versus 103 cm) as well as improvements in blood pressure, triglycerides, blood sugar levels, and insulin sensitivity. In a pilot study, the same dosage of berberine for twelve weeks produced an average weight loss of more than 10 pounds.

2. The white mulberry plant (*Morus alba*) is best known as the food of silkworms, but it is highly regarded in traditional Chinese and Japanese medicine. Recently, human clinical studies have confirmed the benefits of mulberry leaf extract in helping to improve blood sugar control, promote weight loss, and prevent and treat type 2 diabetes as well as combat metabolic syndrome and cardiovascular disease. Many of the effects of mulberry leaf extract are due to its positive influence on AMPk activity. The daily dosage is equivalent to 3,000 mg of dried mulberry leaves. Extracts are generally used. The dosage of a 10:1 extract is 300 mg daily.

3. Another popular dietary weight-loss supplement that activates AMPk is green coffee bean extract. The extract is rich in chlorogenic acid, a compound that has been shown to improve glucose metabolism, inhibit the accumulation of fat, and decrease the absorption of glucose in the intestines. Roasting coffee beans destroys most of the chlorogenic acid, so drinking coffee will not yield these benefits. Only raw green coffee beans contain a significant amount of this health-promoting compound. Clinical studies indicate that green coffee bean extract can promote weight loss, as well as reduce blood pressure in people with hypertension. The typical dosage recommendation is 400 mg three times daily.

The Human Microbiome, Insulin Resistance, and AMPk

The role of gut microorganisms in determining our health is enormous. Just consider that we have more microbial cells in our intestinal tract than we have cells in our entire body. The modern term for our gut flora is "human microbiome." It may be that weight loss could be as simple as making sure a person has the right intestinal flora.

A possible link between gut flora and obesity was first discovered by comparing intestinal bacteria in obese and lean individuals. There were significant differences. That led to studies in animals that found that when skinny mice were inoculated with the bacterial flora of the fat mice, they became fat themselves and vice versa.

Here is what is currently known. Eating a Western-style high-fat, high-sugar diet causes distinct shifts in the microbiome that are associated with insulin resistance, obesity, and type 2 diabetes. Fortunately, shifts in the content of the microbiome can occur rapidly, as human studies have shown that gut microbiome can change considerably in even a day's time.

Particularly important in the health and composition of the microbiome are prebiotics, a general term referring primarily to dietary fiber and other food components that promote the growth and/or activity of microorganisms (bacteria or fungi) that contribute a beneficial effect to the microbiome. Also important to the health of the microbiome are various dietary components that prevent the overgrowth of yeast and harmful bacteria.

A large body of emerging evidence indicates that having the right type of bacteria and yeast in the microbiome plays a significant role in insulin activity, AMPk activation, and satiety. Some of these effects are mediated through the production of metabolic by-products of health-promoting gut bacteria, including short-chain fatty acids. These molecules are the primary energy source for the cells that line the colon and exert significant protective effects against colon cancer.

Probiotics to Promote AMPk Activation, Weight Loss, and Blood Sugar Control

While the focus should be on diet to influence the gut microbiome, probiotics can definitely aid AMPk activation, weight loss, and blood sugar control. "Probiotic" describes the beneficial bacteria that inhabit the human intestinal tract. Probiotics include fermented foods such as yogurt, sauerkraut, and kefir, as well as specific supplements containing freeze-dried bacteria. The specific microorganisms found in these products are usually lactobacilli and bifidobacteria. These bacteria are the major probiotics in the human intestinal tract and show tremendous health benefits. Now some human studies are showing that probiotic supplementation can also promote weight loss.

In a study published in 2014 in the *British Journal of Nutrition*, 125 overweight men and women underwent a twelve-week weight-loss diet, followed by a twelve-week period aimed at maintaining body weight. Throughout the entire study, half the participants took two probiotic capsules daily that provided 3.2 billion colony-forming units (CFUs) of *Lactobacillus rhamnosus*, while the other half took a placebo. After the twelve-week diet period, the women in the study had an average weight loss of 9.7 pounds if they were in the probiotic group and 5.7 pounds if in the placebo group. After the twelve-week maintenance period, the weight of the women in the placebo group had remained stable, but the probiotic group had continued to lose weight, for a total of 11.5 pounds per person. Thus the women consuming the probiotic supplement lost twice as much weight over the twenty-four-week period of the study. Interestingly, no differences in weight loss were observed among the men in the two groups.

A 2011 study conducted at Turku University Hospital in Finland provides some additional food for thought. In the study, 159 pregnant women were randomized to receive either *Lactobacillus rhamnosus* (10 billion CFUs) or a placebo for four weeks before expected delivery and six months postpartum. The children were followed over their first ten years. It was found that this short-term probiotic supplementation had a protective effect against excessive weight gain in the children over the first years of life.

As to how gut bacteria influence weight loss, several mechanisms are now well established. Interestingly, they all impact AMPk. My recommendation is that for the best weight-loss probiotic, it's best to take a multistrain formula to take advantage of the many species associated with positive effects on weight loss. The recommended dosage of a probiotic capsule is 10 to 12 billion CFUs daily.

Throughout *The Magic of Food* you will find additional information on what foods to eat to improve insulin sensitivity, activate AMPk, impact appetite and satiety, and promote a healthy body weight.

Why Dietary Fats Are Essential

We cannot live without fat. Fatty substances perform many vital functions in every cell of the body. Fats are required for the membrane barrier of our body cells; they surround nerves so they can function properly and allow nerve impulses to travel to and from the brain and other organs. Some fats are transformed into hormonelike substances that regulate many body processes, including inflammation, blood flow, and immune function. Other fats act as insulation and cushioning within the body, and fat cells store vital resources.

Dietary fats are often given a bad rap because they are associated with making us fat. Whenever extra dietary calories are consumed in a day, they are converted to body fat and stored in fat cells. Since the human body has an almost unlimited capacity to store fat, eating a diet too high in calories from any source can lead to obesity. Dietary fats are the most concentrated source of calories because they provide 9 calories per gram, compared to 4 calories per gram for carbohydrates and protein. When trying to lose weight, many people cut down their calorie intake by reducing their fat intake.

That's not a good idea, however. It's important to eat healthy fats and avoid those that negatively affect our bodies. In the right form and amount, dietary fats are magical and will help you achieve and maintain your ideal body weight and optimal health.

Fat Nomenclature

Fat molecules are made of carbon, hydrogen, and oxygen atoms. Each of the atoms attaches to the others only in certain predetermined ways. The backbone of a fat is a chain of carbon atoms. Hydrogen and oxygen atoms can then attach to the carbons. A *saturated fat* is a fat molecule in which all of the available binding sites are occupied by another atom. In other words, the carbons are *saturated* with all of the atoms they can hold. An *unsaturated fat* has one or more bonding sites left unoccupied; the two neighboring carbon atoms will take up the slack by forming a double bond, which can be either a *cis* or a *trans* configuration (discussed below).

A fat molecule with one double bond is called a *monounsaturated fat*. Molecules with more than one double bond are called *polyunsaturated fats*. *Mono-* means "one"; *poly-* means "many." When an unsaturated fat contains the first double bond at the third carbon, it is referred to as an omega-3 fatty acid. If the first double bond is at the sixth carbon, it is an omega-6 fatty acid, and if it occurs at the ninth carbon, it is an omega-9 fatty acid.

To illustrate the difference in structure, let's look at the 18-carbon family of fatty acids. Stearic acid is an 18-carbon-long saturated fatty acid, which means that it is carrying as many carbon molecules as it can.

Oleic acid is an 18-carbon-long monounsaturated fatty acid. It is missing two hydrogen molecules, leaving two carbon molecules unsaturated. This causes the carbons to bind to each other to form a double bond. Oleic acid is a monounsaturated fatty acid because it contains one double bond at the ninth carbon molecule. A shorthand way to write this structure is C18:1w9. This means that oleic acid is a fatty acid composed of a chain of 18 carbon molecules and one double bond at the ninth carbon. Oleic acid is an omega-9 fatty acid because its first unsaturated bond occurs at the ninth carbon from the omega end.

Linoleic acid is an 18-carbon-long polyunsaturated fatty acid because it contains two double bonds. Linoleic acid would be written C18:2w6. Linoleic acid is classified as an omega-6 fatty acid as the first double bond occurs at the sixth carbon.

The other essential fatty acid is alpha-linolenic acid. It is also an 18-carbon-long polyunsaturated fatty acid like linoleic acid, but it has three double bonds, written C18:3w3. Alpha-linolenic acid is an omega-3 fatty acid because its first double bond is at the third carbon from the omega end.

Double bonds cause bends in the molecule. It can bend in a cis form, which assumes a horseshoe shape, or a trans shape, to extend the chain.

Most mono- and polyunsaturated fats in nature are in the cis form. As a result, when mono- or polyunsaturated oils are in the cis form they are liquid at room temperature or when refrigerated. In contrast, trans oils such as margarine and shortening are solid or semisolid at room temperature. Margarine and shortening are manufactured from vegetable oils through hydrogenation. This means that a hydrogen molecule is added to the natural unsaturated fatty acid molecules of the vegetable oil to make it more saturated. Hydrogenation, the addition of hydrogen molecules, changes the structure of the natural fatty acid into many unnatural fatty acid forms, as well as from the cis configuration to its mirror image, the trans configuration. The structural changes that occur in the fatty acids in the process of making margarine or shortening carry significant health risks. An overwhelming amount of data has shown that trans fatty acids increase the risk of almost every disease imaginable. They can be found in many foods, especially processed ones. Avoid fried foods such as doughnuts and French fries; baked goods including cakes, pie crusts, biscuits, frozen pizza, cookies, and crackers; and margarines.

EPA and DHA

Two additional members of the omega-3 family deserve special mention: eicosapentaenoic acid (EPA) and docosahexaenoic acid (DHA). These have longer chains than alpha-linolenic acid and have more double bonds as well. EPA is abbreviated 20:5w3, and DHA is 22:6w3.

The reality is that there are tremendous differences in the shapes of fatty acids. That is important because their shape is critical to their structural and physiological effects.

EPA and DHA are the chief omega-3 fatty acids found in cold-water fish and fish oil supplements. EPA and DHA are important as they are transformed into regulatory compounds known as prostaglandins. These compounds act like hormones and carry out many important tasks in the body. Through their effects on prostaglandins and related compounds, long-chain omega-3 fatty acids influence many important biological processes, especially inflammation. As a result, omega-3 fatty acids are useful in the treatment and prevention of almost every chronic disease.

Although it is possible for the body to convert ALA to EPA and DHA, this conversion does not happen efficiently, especially in men. Although the body can convert ALA, a short-chain omega-3 fatty acid, from flaxseed oil, it is more efficient to get preformed EPA and DHA from fish, especially cold-water fish such as salmon, mackerel, herring, and sardines, and taking a fish oil supplement.

What About Meat as a Source of DHA?

Promoters of the paleo diet recommend that we eat as our ancestors did when they were hunters and gatherers, before they began to grow their own food. The best parts of the diet recommend eating more whole foods and avoiding processed foods. One of the other positive aspects of the paleo diet is that it has increased our awareness of how much our food supply has changed due to manufacturing and agrobusiness.

The paleo diet also includes significant amounts of meat—beef, pork, lamb, chicken, turkey, and game. There is an enormous difference between the lean, wild meats our ancestors hunted and consumed and the farm-raised meats we find in today's supermarkets. For example, domesticated animals such as the pig and cow have a much higher fat level than their wild counterparts (25% to 30% or higher fat content in domesticated animals compared to less than 4% for free-living animals or wild game). The type of fat is also considerably different. Domesticated beef, fed a diet of mostly corn and soy, contains saturated fats, omega-6 fatty acids, and virtually undetectable amounts of omega-3 fatty acids. In contrast, wild animals and grass-fed beef contain good amounts of beneficial omega-3 fatty acids (approximately 4%), including DHA, and a much lower omega-6-to-omega-3 ratio (>20:1 in grain-fed beef and about 2:1 to 3:1 in grass-fed beef). So there are significant advantages to eating grass-fed beef.

Why Fatty Acids are Essential

Technically, the only two official essential fatty acids are linoleic (an omega-6 fat) and alpha-linolenic acid (an omega-3 fat). They are considered essential nutrients because the body cannot manufacture them; they must be ingested. Other fats are beneficial but not essential. In this day of fat phobia and the resultant barrage of low-fat and nonfat food products lining the grocery aisles, it is ironic that many experts estimate that approximately 80% of the population consumes an insufficient quantity of essential and health-promoting fatty acids. This dietary insufficiency of essential fats presents a serious health threat.

In general, a deficiency of essential fatty acids can be so vague and broad that symptoms are typically written off as one of myriad other causes. Signs and symptoms typical of, but not exclusive to, essential fatty acid deficiency include:

- Fatigue, malaise, lack of energy and endurance
- Dry skin and hair and cracked nails
- Dry mucous membranes, tear ducts, mouth, and vagina
- Flatulence, bloating, and constipation
- Frequent colds and flulike illnesses
- Sore joints and arthritis
- Chest pain
- Depression, lack of motivation, and forgetfulness
- High blood pressure
- Cardiovascular disease

Measuring Omega-3 Fatty Acids in the Blood

There is a simple blood test that is more significant than cholesterol measurements in determining your risk of having a heart attack or stroke. This same test can predict your risk of Alzheimer's disease, many forms of cancer, and chronic degenerative diseases. It also provides critical information in monitoring and dealing with autism, attention deficit disorder, rheumatoid arthritis, cancer, and more than sixty other conditions and serious illnesses.

The test simply measures the levels of omega-3 fatty acids in the blood. There are several options of tests available directly to consumers. These tests kits contain everything you need to collect a small amount of blood from a simple skin prick of a finger that is placed on a special filter paper and sent to the lab. Your complete results can be emailed or mailed directly to you. The results come complete with an interpretation and recommendations.

The best option for testing is through Grassroots Health. This group is leading an international research initiative for omega-3 fatty acids and vitamin D that will result in even more scientific data on the power of these important nutrients for a wide variety of health conditions. The test kit measures the Omega-3 Index and vitamin D3 levels. The cost is $99.00 plus $5.00 shipping. For more information, go to omega3d.grassrootshealth.net.

Even without the test, know that most people need to lower their intake of omega-6 oils while increasing their intake of omega-3 fats, especially the longer-chain omega-3s EPA and DHA.

Good Fats Versus Bad Fats

What makes a fat "bad" or "good" has to do with two key factors: (1) the way the fatty acids function as structural components in cell membranes and (2) their effect on hormonelike molecules known as eicosanoids.

Cell membranes are made mostly of fatty acids. What determines the type of fatty acid present in the cell membrane is the type of fat you consume. If it is mostly saturated fat and cholesterol from meat and dairy products, the results will be less-than-optimal membranes as opposed to those of people who consume higher levels of monounsaturated and polyunsaturated fatty acids.

Considerable evidence indicates that cell membrane dysfunction makes a person more susceptible to many diseases. Without healthy membranes, cells lose their ability to hold water, vital nutrients, and electrolytes. They also lose their ability to communicate with other cells and to be controlled by regulating hormones, including insulin. Without the right type of fats in cell membranes, cells do not function properly.

Sources of Good Fats and Bad Fats	
Good Fats	**Bad Fats**
Sources of monounsaturated fats:	**Sources of artificial trans fatty acids:**
Nuts and seeds Olive oil Avocado oil Canola oil Macadamia nut oil Sunflower oil (high oleic only)	Partially hydrogenated vegetable oil Shortening Margarine Many baked goods, cookies, icings, crackers, etc. Read food labels carefully.
Sources of alpha-linolenic acid, an omega-3 fatty acid:	**Sources of linoleic acid, an omega-6 fatty acid, and other undesirable oils:**
Flaxseed Flaxseed oil Walnuts Chia seeds Canola oil Soy Sunflower	Most vegetable oils, including: Corn Cotton seed Grape seed Safflower
Sources of EPA and DHA, the longer-chain omega-3 fatty acids:	**Sources of oxidized fats:**
Cold-water fish such as salmon, mackerel, herring, etc. Fish oil supplements	Fried foods Charbroiled meat
Sources of medium-chain saturated fats:	**Sources of longer-chain saturated fats:**
Coconut oil Grass-fed meat and dairy products Organic free-range chicken and eggs Wild salmon	High-fat meat and dairy products Grain- or soy-fed meat and dairy products Conventionally raised chicken and eggs Farmed salmon

Since the kinds of dietary fat consumed determine cell membrane composition, poor fat choices lead to reduced membrane fluidity, which in turn causes reduced insulin binding to receptors on cellular membranes and/or reduced insulin action. The resistance to the hormone insulin is the underlying factor that leads to weight gain, difficulty in losing weight, and the development of obesity and type 2 diabetes. Insulin resistance is also linked to cancer, heart disease, Alzheimer's disease, and many other conditions. Fortunately, we can take steps to reduce the development of these diseases by making sure we eat the right dietary fats.

Olive Oil

The health benefits of olive oil have been mentioned previously. It is one of the key components of the Mediterranean diet. People who consume olive oil regularly, especially in place of other fats, have much lower rates of heart disease, atherosclerosis, diabetes, colon cancer, asthma, and many other diseases.

Technically speaking, the olive is a fruit. The fact that olives are rich in oil is reflected in the botanical name of the olive tree, *Olea europaea*, as *oleum* means "oil" in Latin. Olive oil is made from the crushing and then subsequent pressing of olives.

The only difference between green olives and black olives is their degree of ripeness; unripe olives are green, and fully ripe olives are black. Black olives contain more oil than green ones. Olive oil is available in a variety of grades, which reflect the degree to which it has been processed. Extra-virgin olive oil is the unrefined oil from the first pressing of the fruit; virgin olive oil refers to all oil produced from the first pressing. As far as health benefits go, always choose extra-virgin oil over virgin. The extra-virgin is higher in the "secret ingredients" of olive oil, the polyphenols, and tastes better. It is also lower in free oleic acid levels, so it is less likely to go rancid. Also, make sure you see the term "cold pressed" on the bottle as it means that heat was not used; the oil was pressed mechanically under lower temperatures.

Since olive oil can become rancid from exposure to light and heat, there are some important criteria to follow when purchasing. Look for extra-virgin olive oils sold in dark bottles, which will help protect the oil from oxidation caused by exposure to light. In addition, make sure the oil is displayed in a cool area, away from any direct or indirect contact with heat.

Storing olive oil properly is important, too, not only to preserve the delicate taste of the oil but to ensure that it does not spoil and become rancid, which will have a negative effect on its nutritional profile. Though some people like to keep olive oil in a metal container near the stove, this exposure to heat will expedite spoilage. It is best to store olive oil in a tinted glass container in a dark, cool cupboard. The same is true for the other mono- or polyunsaturated oils. Consume a bottle of olive oil quickly, before it spoils.

Here are some quick serving ideas to gain the health benefits of olive oil:

- Use olive oil in salad dressings.
- Olive oil with herbs and spices makes a great base for marinades for chicken, fish, beef, and soy products such as tofu and tempeh.
- Puree roasted garlic, cooked potatoes, and olive oil together to make delicious garlic mashed potatoes. Season to taste.
- Drizzle olive oil over sautéed vegetables before serving.
- Puree olive oil, garlic, and your favorite beans together in a food processor. Season to taste and serve as a dip or sandwich spread.

Macadamia Nut Oil

The macadamia tree (*Macadamia integrifolia*) is native to the tropical rain forests of Australia. One of the reasons macadamia nuts have such a wonderful flavor is their high fat content (72%). Macadamia nut oil, in my opinion, is the best oil for sautéing and other types of cooking. I would rate avocado oil number two, then olive oil.

Macadamia nut oil is superior to cook with because of its lower level of polyunsaturated fatty acids (3% for macadamia nut oil versus 8% for olive and 23% for canola). Though olive oil and canola oil can form lipid peroxides at relatively low cooking temperatures, macadamia nut oil is stable at much higher temperatures (over twice that of olive oil and four times as stable as canola). Macadamia oil, like olive oil, is also high in natural antioxidants. In fact, it contains more than 4.5 times the amount of vitamin E that olive oil does.

Several studies conducted at the University of Hawaii have shown significant health benefits of macadamia nut oil. It is particularly effective in

lowering total cholesterol and LDL cholesterol concentrations as well as triglyceride levels. Macadamia nut oil is also a great source of a special fatty
acid, palmitoleic acid, which has been shown to increase insulin sensitivity
by suppressing inflammation. You can use macadamia nut oil in recipes in
place of olive oil.

Avocado Oil

Pressed from avocados, this oil is an excellent source of monounsaturated fat
with a smoke point of 500°F versus 320°F for extra-virgin olive oil, making it a
great choice for sautéing. It is also a good choice for dressing salads.

Avocados are also an excellent source of potassium, vitamin E, B vitamins,
and fiber. One avocado has the potassium content of two to three bananas
(about 1,000 mg of potassium). An avocado also has about three times as
many calories as a banana. A 3½-ounce (100-gram) serving is about half an
avocado and provides 160 calories, 2.0 grams of protein, 14.7 grams of fat, 8.5
grams of carbohydrate, and 6.7 grams of fiber.

Avocados contain a moderate level of phytochemicals, especially polyphenols that show antioxidant activity. They have the highest fruit antioxidant
capacity in protecting against the formation of damaged fats (lipid peroxides)
in the blood. Avocados and avocado oil promote healthy blood lipid profiles
and enhance the bioavailability of fat-soluble vitamins and phytochemicals
from other fruits and vegetables. Eating avocados with salads or salsa increases
the bioavailability of carotenoids multifold, which may add to their potential
health benefits.

A total of eight clinical trials have shown the consumption of avocados to
have cardiovascular benefits, including improvements in cholesterol levels. In
subjects with high blood cholesterol levels, avocado-enriched diets improved
blood lipid profiles by lowering LDL cholesterol and triglyceride levels and
increasing HDL cholesterol levels, compared with high-carbohydrate diets or
other diets without avocado.

Along with the benefits to cardiovascular health, several preliminary clinical studies indicate that avocados can support weight control. The avocado's
calories seem to be offset by its ability to make you feel full and satisfied for a

longer period of time than many other foods. In a randomized single-blind, crossover study of twenty-six healthy overweight adults, when the subjects ate half an avocado as part of their lunchtime meal, they reported significantly reduced hunger and increased satiation compared to those who didn't eat avocado at the control meal.

Canadian researchers at Waterloo University identified a compound in avocados, avocatin B, as a substance that causes selective toxicity to the abnormal cells in acute myeloid leukemia (AML). Specifically, their research using functional cell assays showed that avocatin B reduced the viability of AML stem cells without effects on normal stem cells.

Their next step was explaining this effect by discovering the mechanism. What they discovered was that avocatin B was toxic to AML cancer cells because it inhibited the ability of mitochondria, the energy-producing compartment of cells, to utilize fats as an energy source. Basically, the avocatin B turned off the cancer cells, leading to a process known as apoptosis, a type of cellular suicide.

What is exciting about this research is the selectivity of the avocatin B, which had no effect on normal cells. Although a lot more research is obviously required before avocatin B becomes a proven treatment for AML, this line of research is encouraging.

Coconut Oil

Coconut oil is different from the monounsaturated oils, because it contains short- and medium-chain triglycerides. In contrast, the saturated fats in animal products are long-chain triglycerides. Being shorter in length, short- and medium-chain triglycerides are handled by the body differently and are preferentially sent to the liver to be burned as energy. In fact, these fats have been shown to promote weight loss by increasing the burning of calories (thermogenesis), plus some research suggests that they lower cholesterol as well.

Approximately 50% of the fatty acids in coconut oil are in the form of a medium-chain (12-carbon) saturated fat called lauric acid, a health-promoting fat whose only other abundant source in nature is human breast milk. In the body, lauric acid is converted into a beneficial compound called monolaurin, an antiviral, antibacterial, and antiprotozoal monoglyceride that destroys a wide variety of disease-causing organisms.

Coconut oil protects against heart disease and promotes weight loss when it is substituted for other fats in the diet. Coconut's medium-chain fats are easily absorbed and preferentially used as an energy source; their burning actually increases the body's metabolic rate. The result—as long as calories in excess of the body's needs are not consumed—is that more calories are burned, which encourages the burning of the long-chain fatty acids found in other fats as well.

Coconut oil may also help improve energy production within brain cells. Combined with a low-carbohydrate diet, coconut oil may enhance memory and cognition in some people with mild to moderate Alzheimer's disease. It may also help improve control of epileptic seizures.

Cooking with Oils

The best oils to cook with are monounsaturated oils and coconut oil. That said, I would opt for the monounsaturated varieties. Though extra-virgin olive oil and canola oil are popular monounsaturated fats, I like macadamia nut and avocado oils even more. They can be used in place of olive oil whenever desired, including in the recipes provided later in the book. They both create a flavorful effect on the food and have a higher smoke point. In cooking, the smoke point of an oil or fat is the temperature at which it begins to break down to glycerol and free fatty acids and produce bluish smoke. The glycerol is then further broken down to acrolein, a toxic substance that is irritating to the eyes and throat.

Canola oil is made from the rapeseed plant, which has been bred so that a toxic oil, erucic acid, has been removed. It has gained incredible popularity in a short period of time because it is being promoted for its high level (7%) of omega-3 oils.

Another healthy option is high-oleic-acid sunflower oil. It is almost a pure monounsaturated fat. However, neither canola nor high-oleic-acid sunflower oil possesses the other benefits provided by macadamia, avocado, and olive oils because they lack some of the "magical" components (e.g., polyphenols) that these other oils provide. The fatty acid profile is great; they just lack the special factors and as a result do not pack as much of a punch for good health. Definitely go with organic canola oil if you use it, as conventional rapeseed is a heavily sprayed crop and 80% of canola oil is from GMO seed. Look for organic, cold-expeller-pressed brands. The lower-cost products sold in supermarkets are most often extracted with chemical solvents or high-speed presses that generate heat. Both methods alter the oil's fatty acids in undesirable ways.

Smoke Point of Selected "Good" Cooking Oils		
Oils	Smoke Point °C	Smoke Point °F
Avocado oil	271°C	520°F
Canola oil (cold pressed)	204°C	400°F
Coconut oil	177°C	350°F
Macadamia nut oil	199°C	390°F
Olive oil (extra-virgin)	160°C	320°F
Sunflower oil (high-oleic-acid variety)	232°C	450°F

Nuts and Seeds Contain Good Fats

Many people shy away from eating nuts and seeds because they are high in calories. Studies have shown that people who frequently consume nuts have less of a weight problem than those who do not. Regular nut and seed consumption—a handful of walnuts, almonds, chia seeds, or sunflower seeds a day—has also been shown to be protective against heart disease. Studies have also shown that nut consumption is associated with significantly reduced risk of developing type 2 diabetes, even in people who are obese.

Nuts and seeds are rich not only in their nutrient content but in their phytochemical content as well. In addition to fiber components, important phytochemicals in nuts and seeds include protease inhibitors, ellagic acid, and other polyphenols.

Nuts are also the best source of arginine, an amino acid that plays an important role in wound healing, detoxification reactions, immune functions, and the secretion of several hormones, including insulin and growth hormone. Recently, there has been a considerable amount of scientific investigation regarding arginine's role in the formation of nitric oxide. This compound plays a central role in determining the tone of blood vessels. Specifically, it exerts a relaxing effect on blood vessels, thereby improving blood flow. Normally, the body makes enough arginine, even when the diet is lacking. In some instances, however, the body may not be able to keep up with increased requirements, and higher dietary intakes may prove useful. Arginine supplementation has been shown to be beneficial in a number of cardiovascular diseases, including angina pectoris, congestive heart failure, high blood pressure, and peripheral vascular insufficiency (decreased blood flow to the legs or arms). By increasing nitric oxide levels, arginine supplementation improves blood flow, reduces blood clot formation, and improves blood fluidity (the blood becomes less viscous and therefore flows through blood vessels more easily). The degree of improvement offered by arginine supplementation in angina and other cardiovascular diseases can be quite significant due to improved nitric oxide levels. These benefits may also be attained by eating foods high in arginine such as nuts.

Science has shown that nuts have two key effects that help fight obesity: first, they promote satiety, the feeling of appetite satisfaction; second, they increase the action of insulin, thereby improving blood sugar control, appetite regulation, and metabolism.

Though it may seem counterintuitive that a high-calorie food can fight obesity, it has been suggested that nuts may not be as high in absorbable calories as once thought. Researchers have looked at the absorption of almonds as an example. Studies have shown that even after thorough chewing, a high proportion of the fat remains encapsulated in the cells of the chewed almond tissue and is therefore less available for digestion. This effect is easily measured by examining the rise in fats in the blood after consumption of almonds. It is thought that the calorie content of almonds, and perhaps nuts in general, is overestimated by about one-third.

To put this estimation to the test, a study was conducted to quantify the effects of chewing on the bioavailability of calories from almonds and also to examine microstructural physical characteristics of chewed-up (masticated) almonds. In the study, seventeen healthy subjects chewed raw natural almonds (NAs) or roasted almonds (RAs) in four separate sessions. After chewing thoroughly, they spit out the food bolus so that researchers could measure the particle size using mechanical sieving and laser diffraction. The microstructure of masticated almonds, including the structural integrity of the cell walls, was examined with microscopy. The ability to absorb the fat from the almonds was predicted by using a theoretical model, based on particle size and cell dimensions, and then compared with empirically derived data.

Results showed that the bioavailability of fat from the almonds masticated by the human volunteers was approximately 8% and 11% for NAs and RAs, respectively. This low percentage of fat bioavailability is attributable to the high proportion (35% to 40%) of large particles (>500 μm) in masticated almonds. Microstructural examination of the almonds by microscopy indicated that most of the fat remained undisturbed in intact cells after the almonds were thoroughly chewed.

The bottom line is that almonds have a lower calorie content than previously thought because as much as 90% of their fat isn't absorbed. I still recommend keeping the portion size moderate if you are trying to lose weight. If so, eat about ¼ cup or a small handful of nuts and seeds a day to gain their nutritional value.

Flaxseed

Flaxseed oil is an excellent source of both essential fatty acids: alpha-linolenic acid (an omega-3 fatty acid) and linoleic acid (an omega-6 fatty acid). Although the body can convert alpha-linolenic acid, a short-chain omega-3 fatty acid, from flaxseed oil, it is much more efficient to get EPA and DHA from fish oils. Furthermore, there is evidence that many people, particularly many men, have a difficult time converting sufficient amounts of alpha-linolenic acid to EPA and DHA. Also, the long-chain omega-3 fatty acids, but not alpha-linolenic acid, are transformed into prostaglandins (see above). Nonetheless, I do recommend adding flaxseed oil or ground flaxseed to your diet. In fact, flaxseed is one of my top seven superfoods and is discussed fully in chapter 6.

Don't cook with flaxseed oil; it is far too fragile and is easily damaged by heat and light. You can add it to cooked foods or use it as a salad dressing, or you can take a tablespoon daily. You can also add ground flaxseed, sometimes called flaxseed meal, to your diet. Flaxseed can be purchased either whole or already ground or sliced. I prefer purchasing ground/milled flaxseed as grinding enhances its digestibility and therefore its nutritional value. Most of the beneficial research has focused on the use of ground flaxseed.

Purchase ground flaxseed in a vacuum-sealed package. Once opened, refrigerate ground flaxseed since it is prone to oxidation, spoilage, and rancidity. Be sure to refrigerate flaxseed oil as well. Here are some quick ways to get your daily dose of flaxseed:

- Add 1 to 2 tablespoons ground flaxseed to your hot or cold cereal.
- Add 1 to 2 tablespoons ground flaxseed to your breakfast smoothie.
- To give cooked vegetables a nuttier flavor, sprinkle 1 tablespoon ground flaxseed on top of them.
- Mix 1 to 2 tablespoons ground flaxseed into yogurt.

Other Seeds

All seeds are nutritional powerhouses. Those that are especially health promoting are chia, sunflower, and pumpkin seeds. These seeds are widely available and inexpensive, and they are valuable additions to your daily nutrition. In addition to nibbling on ¼ cup seeds as a snack, they can be added to many foods.

- Add chia seeds to smoothies, yogurt, guacamole, hummus, oatmeal, and sauces.
- Sprinkle chia, sunflower, or pumpkin seeds on top of mixed green salads.
- Add pumpkin or sunflower seeds to tuna, chicken, or turkey salad.

Bad Fats: Trans Fats and Other Synthetic Fats

For many years, margarines containing trans fatty acids manufactured from vegetable oils through hydrogenation were promoted as healthy alternatives to butter. They were used in processed foods such as crackers, cookies, baked goods, ice cream, and prepared snack foods. Ultimately, research showed that these synthetic fats are damaging to human health. In 2013, the FDA withdrew their designation as Generally Recognized as Safe (GRAS), and in 2015 it initiated a process to ban the presence of trans fatty acids added to foods by 2018.

In hydrogenation, a hydrogen molecule is added to the natural unsaturated fatty acid molecules of the vegetable oil to make it more saturated or "partially hydrogenated." The structure of the natural fatty acid is thus changed to many "unnatural" fatty acid forms. In most cases the fats are changed from the natural cis configuration to its mirror image, the trans configuration, so that they are solid or semisolid at room temperature.

When ingested, trans fatty acids are incorporated into cell membranes. Trans fat intake is linked to an increased risk of coronary heart disease, some cancers, infertility, and many other serious health issues. By banning the addition of trans fats to foods, the FDA estimates that thousands of fatal heart attacks will be prevented every year.

Other synthetic fats in our food supply are also dangerous. For example, the compound diacetyl is used to give foods a buttery flavor. It is found in many products, including butter-flavored microwave popcorn, cookies, crackers, potato chips, corn chips, margarine, and many more.

A study completed at the University of Minnesota showed that diacetyl potently enhances the ability of a substance known as beta-amyloid to damage or destroy brain cells. As discussed in chapter 1, the formation of beta-amyloid and its resultant effect on destroying brain cells is one of the key underlying factors that contributes to Alzheimer's disease. The takeaway is clear: avoid diacetyl-containing foods if you want to reduce your risk of Alzheimer's disease.

Fats: What to Eat and What to Avoid

This chapter has presented a lot of information to help you create better health by improving the fat content of your body through diet and supplementation. Here are the key points:

1. Be aware of the fat content of foods. Your total daily intake of dietary fats should be no more than 30% of calories consumed (400 to 600 calories a day from fat, based on a 2,000-calorie-a-day diet). Eliminate omega-6 fatty acid sources as much as possible and focus on the "good" fats, particularly monounsaturated fatty acids, coconut oil, and omega-3 fatty acids.

2. Increase the amount of monounsaturated fats in your diet. While most nuts and seeds are relatively high in fat, the calories they supply come mostly from monounsaturated fats. Consume about ¼ to ½ cup or a small handful of nuts and seeds at least every other day.

3. Eat more fish; eat less meat and fewer dairy products. Particularly beneficial are cold-water fish, including wild salmon, mackerel, herring, and halibut, because of their high levels of omega-3 fatty acids. Though almost all fish contain trace amounts of methyl mercury, those most likely to have the lowest levels of methyl mercury are salmon (usually nondetectable levels), cod, mackerel, cold-water tuna, farm-raised catfish, and herring. Swordfish, shark, and some other large predatory fish may contain high levels of methyl mercury, so limit your intake of them to no more than once a week. If you are pregnant or planning to become pregnant, limit such fish to no more than once a month.

4. Take a high-quality fish oil supplement. Highly concentrated fish oil capsules providing long-chain omega-3 fatty acids that are free from lipid peroxides, heavy metals, environmental contaminants, and other harmful compounds are readily available. Today's pharmaceutical-grade fish oil concentrates are so superior to earlier products that they

have literally revolutionized nutritional medicine because of the health benefits they provide. Though there is no official standard for pharmaceutical-grade fish oil, read the label on the bottle to see if the capsules have the following characteristics:

- It should be manufactured in a certified GMP (good manufacturing practices) facility approved for pharmaceutical products as certified by either a government organization or the USP (United States Pharmacopeia).
- It should be manufactured according to pharmaceutical standards that include quality control steps to ensure that the product is free from lipid peroxides, heavy metals, environmental contaminants, and other harmful compounds.
- It must provide at least a 60% concentration of the most active long-chain omega-3 fatty acids (EPA and DHA).

If you are a vegetarian or a vegan, there are now algae-based EPA+DHA supplements on the market.

When using fish oil or algae-based supplements, the dosage recommendation for any form is based not on the amount of total fish or algal oil but rather on the amount of EPA and DHA combined. For example, the front label may say 1,000 mg of fish oil per capsule, but the Supplement Facts panel may say that it provides only 180 mg of EPA and 120 mg of DHA for a total of 300 mg of EPA+DHA. So read labels carefully. For general health, the dosage recommendation is 1,000 mg per day of EPA+DHA; for more therapeutic purposes, such as reducing inflammation, lowering triglycerides, or improving brain function and/or mood, the dosage recommendation is 3,000 mg per day of EPA+DHA.

5. Consume 1 tablespoon flaxseed oil or 2 tablespoons ground flaxseed daily. Purchase flaxseed oil in opaque bottles to limit oxidation, and refrigerate after opening. Buy ground flaxseed in a vacuum-sealed package to ensure freshness, and refrigerate after opening.

Dietary Fat and the Human Brain

A larger, more metabolically active brain is one of the key differences between humans and other primates. Some evolutionists have theorized that a shift in the dietary intake of fats was the likely stimulus for brain growth in ancient humans. The shift itself may have been the result of limited food availability, forcing early humans to collect shellfish and hunt grazing mammals, such as antelope and gazelle, in addition to gathering plant foods. Archaeological data support this association. Human brains started to grow and become more developed at about the same time that evidence shows an increase of shellfish consumption and the presence of animal bones being butchered with stone tools. Data also show that the early humans who lived near water sources and ate seafood experienced the most significant changes in the size and development of their brains. An increased intake of the omega-3 fatty acid docosahexaenoic acid (DHA), found primarily in fish and seafood, as well as wild game, was perhaps the largest dietary contributor to brain growth.

The thinking is that a higher DHA intake led to larger human brains. With their larger brains, early humans were able to engage in more complex social behaviors, which led to improved foraging and hunting tactics and even higher-quality food intake, fostering additional brain evolution. In contrast, inland prehistoric man did not have sufficient access to DHA, and Neanderthals ate larger animals with low DHA content. As a result, both humans and animals died off due to limited brain capacity and other factors.

The importance of DHA to brain function relates to its role in the composition of brain cell membranes; it influences:

- The fluidity of brain cell membranes
- Neurotransmitter synthesis
- Neurotransmitter binding
- Signal transmission
- The activity of key enzymes that break down neurotransmitters such as serotonin, epinephrine, dopamine, and norepinephrine.

Specifically, two-thirds of the brain's dry weight comes from fats. It is now known that 60% of the brain's fats are omega-3 fatty acids, DHA being the main type. Cold-water fatty fish are the best source of preformed DHA.

A higher intake of DHA during pregnancy and early childhood was especially important to human evolution. DHA is critical for healthy brain development, both in the womb and in early childhood. About 75% of brain cells are in place before birth, and the other 25% are in place by the age of one year, making DHA an essential nutrient for both pregnant mothers and young children. DHA is so essential for early brain development that it is now often added to baby formula. Pregnant women should also strive to get sufficient levels by regularly eating fish or taking fish oil supplements.

Proper brain and nerve function also require the monounsaturated fat oleic acid, the main component of olive oil, also found in almonds, pecans, macadamias, peanuts, and avocados. Myelin, the protective sheath that covers communicating neurons, is composed of 30% protein and 70% fat, with oleic acid the key fat. Eating high-quality fats can have positive effects on the brain.

A diet including DHA equipped primitive humans with a better-functioning brain, enabling them to survive and flourish. There is substantial data showing that increasing EPA and DHA intake provides considerable health benefits, especially relating to brain function. Keep in mind that DHA is the most abundant fat in the brain and loss of DHA concentrations in brain cell membranes leads to poor brain cell function. Thus, higher intakes of EPA and DHA are associated not only with higher intelligence but also with improved mood and social function. Studies have found that the children of mothers who ate fish on a regular basis (at least once per week) while pregnant have better social and verbal skills at age 8 compared to the children of mothers who never ate fish.

Breastfed infants have higher IQs than formula-fed infants. The availability of DHA in breast milk is one of the key reasons. In a detailed analysis of twenty published studies, researchers at the University of Kentucky showed that the nutritional benefits of breastfeeding are associated with at least a 3.2-IQ-point difference in cognitive development and a 2.1-point increase in maternal bonding. The enhanced cognitive development was seen as early as six months and was sustained through age 15. The longer a baby was breast-fed, the greater the increase in cognitive developmental benefit.

For non-breastfed infants, it is important to choose infant formulas including DHA. According to a 2000 study funded by the National Institute of Child Health and Human Development, adding DHA to infant formula significantly boosts children's average intelligence scores.

A worthwhile goal is helping children get a head start in life by making sure that their brains have all the important nutrients and building blocks they need to develop properly—including DHA. Sadly, low levels of DHA during fetal and infant brain development may be one of the critical reasons why we are seeing so many children on psychoactive drugs for attention deficit disorder, depression, obsessive-compulsive disorder, and other psychological illnesses.

Omega-3 Fatty Acids in Dyslexia, ADD/ADHD, and Dyspraxia

There has been research showing that EPA and DHA may play a role in helping to prevent or treat conditions affecting children's brains such as dyslexia, ADHD (attention-deficit/hyperactivity disorder), and dyspraxia (quality of movement). Numerous studies show that children with low levels of these omega-3 fats can have a decreased ability to focus their attention, which can lead to problems in performing skilled movements, detecting facial and emotional expressions, and sequencing letters and numbers. Studies have shown that fish oil supplements rich in EPA and DHA may help improve the reading skills and attention span of children suffering from dyslexia and ADHD and may also improve motor skills and general coordination. The benefits of omega-3 fats have been seen across many conditions affecting learning in children.

Omega-3 Fatty Acids in Alzheimer's Disease and Dementia

EPA and DHA may contribute to preventing Alzheimer's disease, a condition that now affects an estimated 42% of people over the age of 85 and many younger people as well. Although Alzheimer's disease may have many causes, research suggests that diet in general, and fish consumption in particular, may play an important role. Researchers have found that the brains of patients with Alzheimer's disease have lower levels of EPA and DHA than those of people without Alzheimer's.

A study conducted in Sweden found that people with the highest blood levels of DHA had a 47% lower risk of developing dementia and a 39% lower risk of developing Alzheimer's than people with the lowest levels of DHA. This study suggests that eating fish two to three times a week may help reduce the risk of developing Alzheimer's or dementia by nearly 40%. In other words, out of ten people who develop Alzheimer's disease, four people would not have developed the condition if they had consumed fish two to three times per week or taken the equivalent amount of DHA (and EPA) in the form of a fish oil supplement.

What all the data tells us is that mental decline in old age may not be as inevitable as we think. Several studies have shown that what we eat may have as big an impact on our brains as it does on our hearts and waistlines. Eating plenty of fresh fruits and vegetables seems to be vital in protecting the brain into old age, but just as important is regularly eating fish or taking fish oil supplements.

Omega-3 Fatty Acids and Depression

Depression is among the leading causes of disability worldwide, affecting an estimated 121 million people. There has been a great deal of research into potential nutritional causes of and treatments for depression, but the most promising results come from studies into fish and omega-3 fatty acids. Low levels of EPA+DHA in the body are associated with a greater risk of developing depression. Studies have also reported that countries with high rates of fish oil consumption have low rates of depressive disorder. In addition, there is now increasing evidence that taking supplemental EPA+DHA is quite helpful in the treatment of depression. The effects can be seen as early as two weeks after beginning supplementation (the recommended dosage is 3,000 mg of EPA+DHA daily).

Omega-3 Fatty Acids and Borderline Personality Disorder

Borderline personality disorder (BPD) is characterized by a pervasive pattern of instability of interpersonal relationships, self-image, and mood, as well as marked impulsivity, beginning by early adulthood. In a couple of studies, fish oil supplementation has shown to be effective in improving BPD. For example, in one study, thirty women with BPD were given either 1 gram of EPA or a placebo for eight weeks. Detailed analyses using sophisticated measures found EPA to be superior to placebo in diminishing aggression as well as the severity of depressive symptoms. The authors of the study went so far as to conclude that EPA may be a safe and effective form of primary therapy for women with moderately severe borderline personality disorder.

The significance of this study is profound, given that an estimated six million people in the United States are believed to suffer from symptoms of BPD. All told, this disorder touches an estimated thirty-six million lives, counting spouses and children. If fish oil supplementation can help BPD, it would be a godsend to many.

Other Benefits of Omega-3 Fatty Acids

Though most Americans eat way too many saturated fats and the omega-6 oils found in meats and most vegetable oils, they suffer from a deficiency of the omega-3 oils. This deficiency is associated with an increased risk of developing heart disease and about sixty other conditions, including cancer, arthritis, stroke, high blood pressure, skin diseases, and diabetes. It is estimated that individuals with a higher dietary intake of EPA and DHA reduce their risk of heart disease by roughly 47% compared to individuals with a lower intake. In addition, scientists now know that fish oil consumption can lower the risk of developing many cancers (particularly breast, prostate, colon, and lung cancer) and many other chronic diseases, including Alzheimer's disease, asthma, depression, diabetes, high blood pressure, macular degeneration, multiple sclerosis, and rheumatoid arthritis.

One of the primary areas of focus with omega-3 fatty acids is in preventing cardiovascular disease (CVD). Supplementation with EPA+DHA has little effect on cholesterol levels but does lower triglyceride levels significantly, as well as producing myriad additional beneficial effects, including reduced blood clot formation; improved function of the lining of blood vessels and arterial flexibility; improved blood and oxygen supply to the heart; and a mild effect in lowering blood pressure.

The levels of EPA and DHA within red blood cells have been shown to be highly significant predictors of heart disease. This has been termed the omega-3 index. An omega-3 index of 8% is associated with the greatest protection, whereas an index of 4% is associated with the least. Researchers have determined that eating approximately two 6- to 8-ounce servings of fish per week or taking a fish oil supplement daily with a total of 800 to 1,000 mg of EPA+DHA is required to achieve or surpass the 8% target.

For lowering triglycerides, the dosage for EPA+DHA is much greater, at least 3,000 mg per day, as lower dosages are not effective. Dosages of 3,000 to 4,000 mg of EPA+DHA per day from fish oil supplements typically lower triglyceride levels by 27% to 30% after one month of supplementation.

EPA and DHA Levels in Vegans and Vegetarians

As humans, we all have some basic and essential nutritional needs, whether we choose to be omnivores, vegetarians, or vegans. Vegetarians and vegans are known to have low levels of EPA and DHA. Based upon a new analysis of the fatty acid profiles in vegetarians and vegans, supplementation with marine algae sources seems essential.

The main omega-3 fatty acid in the vegetarian diet is alpha-linolenic acid (ALA), which is derived from foods such as flaxseed and walnuts, as well as their oils. Though some ALA is converted to EPA, it is a rather inefficient conversion, and supplementation with ALA from flaxseed oil has little effect on raising DHA levels.

Based upon a considerable body of evidence, the health benefits of EPA+DHA appear when the concentration within red blood cells achieves a value greater than 8%. Levels under 4% are considered high risk for more than sixty different health conditions. Previous studies have shown that vegans and vegetarians, as well as omnivores who do not eat fish or take fish oil supplements, are typically below 4% of EPA+DHA in their blood.

A study was conducted to better define the level of these omega-3 fatty acids in vegans and to determine the effects on blood measurements of a vegan omega-3 supplement from marine algae providing 254 mg of EPA+DHA a day for four months.

A total of 165 vegans participated in the study. A subset of 46 subjects with a baseline omega-3 index of <4% was given a vegetarian omega-3 supplement for four months and then retested. The average level of EPA+DHA in the blood of the 165 vegans was 3.7%, with roughly two out of three vegans having levels below 4% and one out of three even lower, at less than 3%. These results clearly show that a substantial number of vegans have low omega-3 status.

In the subset that received the marine microalgae–derived EPA+DHA supplement, blood levels increased from 3.1% to 4.8%. These results indicate that although there was a good response to the relatively low dose of EPA+DHA given, higher dosages are required to achieve the target of 8% in these individuals. Again, a total of 800 to 1,000 mg of EPA+DHA daily is required to achieve or surpass the 8% target of the omega-3 index.

Fat consumption, in general, is not the problem. The problem is the excess consumption of so much bad fat. It's time to realize that our bodies and brains need good fats for our health and well-being.

5

The Power of Plant Pigments

One of my major dietary recommendations is for people to consume a "rainbow" of foods, which means a wide range of fruits and vegetables—red tomatoes and strawberries, orange citrus and mangoes, yellow squash and lemons, green kale and broccoli, blueberries and blackberries, and violet beets. These colorful foods provide the body with powerful antioxidant effects as well as the nutrients it needs for optimal function and protection against disease.

Fruits and vegetables are so important in the battle against cancer that some experts posit that cancer is a result of a "maladaptation" over time to a reduced level of intake of fruits and vegetables. As a study published in the medical journal *Cancer Causes and Control* put it, "Vegetables and fruits contain the anticarcinogenic cocktail to which we are adapted. We abandon it at our peril."

When I first started studying nutrition in the late 1970s, the American Cancer Society claimed that there was no link between diet and most cancers. Then, in 1982, the National Academy of Sciences of the United States published a report on diet and cancer, emphasizing the importance of fruits and vegetables. The value of adding citrus fruits, carotene-rich fruits and vegetables, and cruciferous vegetables to the diet for reducing the risk of certain cancers was specifically noted.

This scientific view, shared with consumers in a 1989 report from the National Academy of Sciences, recommended that Americans consume five or more servings of fruits and vegetables daily to reduce the risk of cancers and heart disease. The Five-a-Day program was developed as a tool to increase public awareness of the health benefits of fruit and vegetable consumption, but most Americans come nowhere near this level of intake.

We also know that five servings per day of fruits and vegetables is nowhere near the ideal. The 2010 Dietary Guidelines for Americans recommended, based on a 2,000-calorie diet, that people should eat at least nine servings of fruits and vegetables per day, four of fruits and five of vegetables.

Another 2010 study found that the average consumption of fruits and vegetables in the United States is only 3.6 servings (1.4 of fruits and 2.2 of vegetables) per person per day. The statistics would have been even worse if the study had eliminated commercial fruit juice and potatoes from the tally.

I recommend trying to eat seven servings of vegetables and two to three servings of fruits every day. A serving is loosely defined as 1 cup uncooked or ½ cup cooked vegetable or fruit. Here are some tips to help you eat your daily quota of fruits and vegetables.

- Buy many different kinds of fruits and vegetables, so you have plenty of choices.
- Wash, dry, peel, and cut fruits and vegetables when you bring them home from the market so they're ready to eat.
- Stock up on bags of frozen vegetables for easy cooking.
- For a fruit sundae, layer a bowl with cut-up fruit, vanilla yogurt, shredded coconut, and a handful of nuts.
- Pack a piece of fruit or some cut-up vegetables in your briefcase or backpack.
- Add fruits and vegetables to lunch by having them in soup, salad, or cut up raw.
- Add thinly sliced pears or apples to an omelet.
- Double up on vegetable portions.
- Add dark, leafy greens such as Swiss chard, collards, spinach, or beet greens to stir-fries.

- Choose fresh fruit for dessert. Make a fruit parfait with low-fat yogurt or sherbet topped with berries.
- Add extra vegetables when you prepare soups, sauces, and casseroles. For example, add grated carrots and zucchini to spaghetti sauce.
- Use vegetable-based sauces such as marinara sauce and juices such as low-sodium V8 or tomato juice.

Eat Seven Servings of Vegetables Daily

In Latin, the word for "vegetable" (*olus*) means "to enliven or animate." There is no question that vegetables give us life and are an essential component of any healthful diet. They provide the broadest range of nutrients of any food group and are rich sources of vitamins, minerals, and carbohydrates. Vegetables also provide high quantities of anticancer phytochemicals and various pigments, especially carotenes.

I recommend eating raw as well as cooked vegetables. Certain compounds are available only in raw vegetables, while other nutrients are better absorbed once cooked. When cooking vegetables, err on the side of undercooking; overcooking will result in the loss of important nutrients and change the flavors. Steam, roast, bake, or stir-fry vegetables for the best results. If fresh vegetables are unavailable, frozen vegetables are preferred over their canned counterparts. The only exception is tomato products, such as tomato sauce and paste, because these products provide more absorbable lycopene than raw tomatoes.

I have divided vegetables into three categories: green leafy and cruciferous vegetables; carotene- and flavonoid-rich vegetables; and other vegetables. I want to encourage you to eat a variety of these life-giving foods.

The Three Vegetable Categories

Green leafy and cruciferous vegetables: 2 to 4 servings daily

Alfalfa sprouts

Beet greens

Bok choy

Broccoli

Brussels sprouts

Cabbage

Cauliflower

Chard

Chinese cabbage

Collard greens

Dandelion

Endive

Escarole

Kale

Lettuce (the darker, the better)

Mustard greens

Parsley

Spinach

Turnip greens

Watercress

Carotene- and flavonoid-rich vegetables: 2 to 3 servings daily

Beets

Bell peppers

Carrots

Eggplant

Summer squash

Winter squash, such as acorn
or butternut

Yams or sweet potatoes

Zucchini

Other vegetables: 2 to 3 servings daily

Artichoke (1 medium)

Asparagus

Bean sprouts

Celery

Cucumbers

Fennel

Green or yellow beans

Mushrooms

Okra

Onions

Peas

Radishes

Rhubarb

Rutabaga

Tomatoes, tomato paste,
tomato sauce, tomato juice,
and vegetable juice cocktail

Eat Two to Three Servings of Fruits Daily

While fruits are rich in fiber, antioxidants, and phytochemicals that provide considerable beneficial health effects, they also contain natural sugars that can potentially stress blood sugar control. The table below lists fruit in ascending order in terms of their glycemic load, which reflects their effect on blood sugar levels. Focus on low-glycemic choices. Limit consumption to a total glycemic load no greater than 15 for any three-hour period. In other words, if you hit a glycemic load of 15 with fruit consumption, it means that no other carbohydrate source can be consumed for three hours.

Note: With dried fruit, it is important to limit the serving size in order not to stress blood sugar control.

Fruits by Glycemic Load		
Fruit	Serving Size	Glycemic Load
Plum	66 g (1 fruit)	1.7
Peach	98 g (1 medium)	2.2
Grapefruit	123 g (½ fruit)	2.8
Strawberries	152 g (1 cup)	3.6
Sweet cherries, raw	117 g (1 cup)	3.7
Kiwifruit, with skin	76 g (1 fruit)	5.2
Apple, with skin	138 g (1 medium)	6.2
Grapes	92 g (1 cup)	6.5
Papaya	140 g (1 cup)	6.6
Pears	166 g (1 medium)	6.9
Orange	140 g (1 fruit)	7.2
Watermelon	152 g (1 cup)	7.2
Cantaloupe	177 g (1 cup)	7.8
Apricot, dried	65 g (½ cup)	11.5
Pineapple, raw	155 g (1 cup)	11.9
Banana	118 g (1 medium)	12.2
Mango	165 g (1 cup)	12.8
Prunes	65 g (½ cup)	17.1
Raisins	43 g (small box)	20.5

Should people with diabetes and other blood sugar issues avoid fruit because it's sweet? Not at all! It's all about eating the right types of fruits to help blood sugar control.

Studies that examined the association between individual fruits or fruit groups and total fruit consumption in type 2 diabetes provide some good guidelines. In one of the most detailed studies on the subject, researchers from the Harvard University School of Public Health examined dietary data from 66,105 women from the Nurses' Health Study I; 85,104 women from the Nurses' Health Study II; and 36,173 men from the Health Professionals Follow-up Study. These subjects were free of major chronic diseases when these studies began.

When the researchers looked at the risk of developing diabetes and the consumption of three whole fruit servings per week of different fruits, they found the following risk levels:

26% reduced risk for those eating blueberries

12% reduced risk for those eating grapes and raisins

7% reduced risk for those eating apples and pears

5% reduced risk for those eating bananas

5% reduced risk for those eating grapefruit

10% increased risk for those eating cantaloupe

The risk of developing diabetes for those eating peaches, plums, apricots, prunes, oranges, and strawberries was neutral. In other words, eating these fruits neither increased nor decreased the risk of type 2 diabetes. When the impact of eating three servings of these fruits was compared with drinking the same amount of fruit juice per week, they were shown to be significantly protective. In other words, switching out fruit juice for whole fruit significantly reduced the risk for diabetes (7% lower risk overall for any whole fruit and as much as 33% lower risk for blueberries).

Another takeaway from the above study is to avoid consumption of commercial fruit juices. Many of the beneficial compounds in fruit are destroyed during pasteurization. Fresh (preferably organic) fruit juices retain these beneficial compounds and provide considerable health benefits, but still need to be consumed in limited amounts to maintain proper blood sugar levels. You should drink no more than 6 to 8 ounces per three-hour period and no more than two servings daily.

Phytochemicals: What Makes Fruits and Vegetables Magical

There are many substances in fruits and vegetables that are known to protect against cancer, heart disease, and other chronic diseases. These compounds are collectively referred to as phytochemicals and include a wide range of different types of molecules. Among the most important groups of phytochemicals are pigments such as chlorophyll, carotenes, and flavonoids, found in a rainbow assortment of fruits and vegetables. Other phytochemicals include dietary fiber, enzymes, volatile oils, and vitaminlike compounds.

Although phytochemicals work in harmony with essential nutrients such as vitamin C, vitamin E, B vitamins, zinc, and selenium, they exert considerably greater protection. Many different phytochemicals exert antioxidant activity. An antioxidant is a substance that protects against oxidative damage. The cells of the human body are constantly under attack by free radicals and pro-oxidants. A free radical is a molecule that contains a highly reactive unpaired electron that can bind to cellular molecules and destroy their structure, while a pro-oxidant is a molecule that can damage cell molecules, causing them to interact negatively with oxygen. Just as oxygen can rust iron, when toxic oxygen molecules attack our cells, free-radical or oxidative damage occurs.

Where do these sinister agents come from? Most of the free radicals zipping through our bodies are produced during normal and necessary metabolic processes such as energy generation, detoxification reactions, and immune defense mechanisms. Ironically, the major source of free-radical and oxidative damage in the body is the oxygen molecule—the factor that gives us life is also the one that can do the most harm! Oxidative and free-radical damage is a major cause of aging and is also linked to the development of cancers, heart disease, cataracts, Alzheimer's disease, arthritis, and other chronic degenerative diseases.

Some Examples of Anticancer Phytochemicals		
Phytochemical	**Actions**	**Examples of Sources**
Carotenoids	• Act as antioxidants • Enhance immune functions	Dark-colored vegetables such as carrots, squash, spinach, kale, tomatoes, yams, and sweet potatoes; fruits such as cantaloupe, apricots, and citrus fruits
Coumarin	• Has antitumor properties • Enhances immune functions • Stimulates antioxidant mechanisms	Carrots, celery, fennel, beets, citrus fruits
Dithiolthiones, glucosinolates, and thiocyanates	• Block cancer-causing compounds from damaging cells • Enhance detoxification	Cabbage-family vegetables—broccoli, brussels sprouts, kale, etc.
Flavonoids	• Act as antioxidants • Have direct antitumor effects • Have immune-enhancing properties	Fruits, particularly darker fruits such as berries, cherries, and citrus fruits; also tomatoes, peppers, and greens; legumes
Isoflavonoids	• Block estrogen receptors	Soy and other legumes
Lignans	• Act as antioxidants • Modulate hormone receptors	Flaxseed and flaxseed oil; whole grains, nuts, and seeds
Limonoids	• Enhance detoxification • Block carcinogens	Citrus fruits, celery
Polyphenols	• Act as antioxidants • Block carcinogen formation • Modulate hormone receptors	Green tea, chocolate, red wine
Sterols	• Block production of carcinogens • Modulate hormone receptors	Soy, nuts, seeds

Protection Against Free-Radical Damage

Although the generation of free radicals within the body is significant, it is the environment that contributes greatly to the free-radical load of an individual. Cigarette smoking, for example, greatly increases an individual's free-radical load. Many of the harmful effects of smoking are related to the high levels of free radicals being inhaled, depleting key antioxidant nutrients such as vitamin C and beta-carotene. Other external sources of free radicals include ionizing radiation, chemotherapeutic drugs, air pollutants, pesticides, anesthetics, aromatic hydrocarbons, fried foods, solvents, alcohol, and formaldehyde. These compounds stress the body's antioxidant mechanisms. People exposed to these environmental factors need the additional nutritional support that fresh fruits and vegetables provide.

Antioxidants and enzymes in the plant foods we consume protect our cells against free-radical and oxidative damage. The major antioxidants include vitamins C and E, but the phytochemicals provide an even wider range than these sorts of nutrient antioxidants. Examples of phytochemicals with significant antioxidant activity include polyphenols, flavonoids, carotenes, and sulfur-containing compounds in cabbage-family vegetables. Free radicals must be broken down by enzymes or be chemically neutralized by antioxidants before they react with cellular molecules. Examples of the free radical–scavenging enzymes produced by the body are catalase, superoxide dismutase, and glutathione peroxidase. Taking these enzymes as oral supplements has not been shown to increase enzyme tissue levels. However, ingesting antioxidant nutrients such as manganese, sulfur-containing amino acids, and vitamin C as well as carotenes, flavonoids, and polyphenols has been shown to increase tissue concentrations of the enzymes.

The other way cells can protect themselves against free-radical or oxidative damage is through chemical neutralization via antioxidants binding to the free radical or pro-oxidant. For example, dietary antioxidants block free-radical damage by chemically reacting with the free radical or pro-oxidant to neutralize it. Ingesting rich sources of antioxidant phytochemicals from fresh juices can increase tissue concentrations of these compounds, thereby supporting normal protective mechanisms and blocking free-radical and oxidative damage to cells of the body.

The Rainbow Assortment of Fruits and Vegetables				
Red	Orange	Yellow and Light Green	Dark Green	Blue/Purple
Apples (red)	Apricots	Apples (green or yellow)	Artichoke	Beets
Bell peppers (red)	Bell peppers (orange)	Avocados	Asparagus	Blackberries
Cherries	Butternut squash	Bananas	Bell peppers (green)	Blueberries
Cranberries	Cantaloupe	Bell peppers (yellow)	Broccoli	Cabbage (purple)
Grapefruit	Carrots	Bok choy	Brussels sprouts	Currants
Grapes (red)	Mangoes	Cabbage	Chard	Eggplant
Plums (red)	Oranges	Cauliflower	Collard greens	Grapes (purple)
Radishes	Papaya	Celery	Cucumber	Onions (red)
Raspberries	Pumpkin	Fennel	Green beans	Pears (red)
Strawberries	Sweet potatoes	Kiwifruit	Grapes (green)	Plums (purple)
Tomatoes	Yams	Lemons	Honeydew melons	
Watermelon		Lettuce (light green types)	Kale	
		Limes	Leeks	
		Onions	Lettuce (dark green types)	
		Pears (green or yellow)	Mustard greens	
		Pineapple	Peas	
		Squash (yellow)	Spinach	
		Zucchini	Turnip greens	

The Three Major Pigments: Chlorophyll, Carotenoids, and Flavonoids

Chlorophyll

All life is made possible by the magic of chlorophyll, the green pigment found in the chloroplast compartment of plant cells. It is in the chloroplast that electromagnetic energy (light) is converted to chemical energy in the process known as photosynthesis. The chlorophyll molecule is essential for this reaction to occur.

The natural chlorophyll found in green plants is fat soluble. Most chlorophyll products found in health stores, however, contain water-soluble chlorophyll. In order to produce water-soluble chlorophyll, the natural chlorophyll molecule must be altered chemically. The fat-soluble form, the natural form of chlorophyll as found in green vegetables and other plants, offers several advantages over water-soluble chlorophyll. This statement is particularly true with regard to chlorophyll's ability to stimulate hemoglobin and red blood cell production. It is interesting to note that the chlorophyll molecule in a plant is similar to the heme portion of the hemoglobin molecule of our red blood cells.

Green leafy vegetables are of great benefit to everyone, but especially those with any kind of anemia. These vegetables contain natural fat-soluble chlorophyll as well as other important nutrients, including iron and folic acid.

Carotenoids

Carotenoids include two types of molecules: carotenes and xanthophylls. These pigments range in color from red to yellow in fat-soluble plant pigments. All organisms, whether bacteria or plants, that rely on the sun for energy contain carotenoid molecules. These compounds, via their antioxidant effects, play a crucial role in protecting the organism against damage during the process of photosynthesis, the process of converting sunlight into chemical energy. Basically, carotenoids keep the plant or bacteria cells from being burned by the sun and process of photosynthesis.

In humans, carotenoids play two primary roles. Some carotenes are converted into vitamin A, and all of them exert antioxidant activity. Of the six hundred carotenes that have been identified, about thirty to fifty are believed to have vitamin A activity. Carotenes that the body can convert to vitamin A are referred to as provitamin A carotenes. The best known of this group are beta-carotene and alpha-carotene. Some of the better-known carotenoids without provitamin A activity, but with high antioxidant activity, are lutein, lycopene, zeaxanthin, and astaxanthin.

Preliminary and experimental studies suggest that a higher dietary intake of carotenes provides protection against developing certain cancers (lung, skin, uterine, cervix, gastrointestinal tract, etc.), heart disease, macular degeneration, cataracts, and other health conditions linked to oxidative or free-radical damage. Again, lutein, zeaxanthin, and lycopene appear to offer the greatest benefits.

Carotenoids are found in all plant foods. In general, the greater the intensity of color, the higher the level of carotenes. In green leafy vegetables, beta-carotene is the predominant carotene. Orange-colored fruits and vegetables—carrots, apricots, mangoes, yams, squash—are excellent sources of beta-carotene, but in most plant foods, other provitamin A carotenes typically predominate.

Yellow vegetables have higher concentrations of xanthophylls, but these compounds, including lutein and zeaxanthin, have significant health benefits due to their antioxidant effects.

The red and purple vegetables and fruits, such as tomatoes, red cabbage, berries, and plums contain a large number of non-vitamin-A-active carotenes, such as lycopene, that also have health benefits.

Legumes, grains, and seeds are also significant sources of carotenes. Carotenoids are also found in some animal foods, such as salmon and some other fish, egg yolks, shellfish, milk, and poultry. Good supplemental forms of mixed carotenoids include palm oil carotene products, algal products, carrot oil, and some "green drinks," such as dehydrated barley greens or wheatgrass.

Selected Carotenoids: Vitamin A Activity and Food Sources		
Carotenoid	**Vitamin A Activity (%)**	**Food Sources**
Beta-carotene	100	Green plants, carrots, sweet potatoes, squash, spinach, apricots, green peppers
Alpha-carotene	50–54	Green plants, carrots, squash, corn, watermelons, green peppers, potatoes, apples, peaches
Gamma-carotene	42–50	Carrots, sweet potatoes, corn, tomatoes, watermelons, apricots
Beta-zeacarotene	20–40	Corn, tomatoes, yeast, cherries
Cryptoxanthin	50–60	Corn, green peppers, persimmons, papayas, lemons, oranges, prunes, apples, apricots, paprika, poultry
Lycopene	0	Tomatoes, carrots, green peppers, apricots, pink grapefruit
Zeaxanthin	0	Spinach, paprika, corn, fruits
Lutein	0	Green plants, corn, potatoes, spinach, carrots, tomatoes, fruits
Canthaxanthin	0	Mushrooms, trout, crustaceans
Crocetin	0	Saffron
Capsanthin	0	Red peppers, paprika
Astaxanthin	0	Salmon, algae, red trout, shrimp, crab lobster

Astaxanthin: A Special Carotenoid

Astaxanthin is a deep vibrant red xanthophyll that is found predominantly in marine life, with microalgae the richest source. When microalgae are consumed by salmon, lobster, shrimp, krill, and other sea life, the intense red pigmentation results in these animals having red or pink flesh or outer shells and skins.

Astaxanthin is critical to the survival of these organisms. It is required by microalgae to protect it from damage produced during photosynthesis. Young salmon die or do not develop properly without sufficient astaxanthin in their diet. Astaxanthin also provides protection for some animals by making them less visible in deep water, where the red segment of the spectrum of visible light does not penetrate. The red pigment also plays a role in mating and spawning behavior.

Yes, astaxanthin has antioxidant activity and can definitely help prevent the oxidative damage that contributes to conditions such as aging, insulin resistance, cardiovascular disease, and neurodegenerative conditions such as Alzheimer's disease. And, yes, so do many other natural antioxidants. But astaxanthin is a bit different as an antioxidant and exerts some additional benefits to protect cells.

First, in regard to general antioxidant effects in protecting cell membranes, astaxanthin is more than sixty-five times as powerful as vitamin C, fifty times as powerful as beta-carotene, and ten times as powerful as vitamin E. Second, one of the unique aspects of astaxanthin relates to its size. It is considerably larger and longer than other carotenes. Its size and physical form allow it to be incorporated into cell membranes, where it can span their entire thickness. This enables it not only to protect the inner and outer cell membranes from oxidative damage but also to stabilize them.

Astaxanthin also exerts some specific anti-inflammatory effects that make it quite useful in protecting brain and vascular cells from damage. Since it effectively protects the membrane system of mitochondria (the energy compartment of cells), it can help boost cellular energy production.

More than fifty clinical and experimental studies have shown astaxanthin as a dietary supplement to be potentially helpful in the following conditions:

- Cardiovascular health. Protects the vascular lining, promotes improved blood flow, and keeps LDL cholesterol from becoming oxidized (damaged).

- Eye health. Protects against eye fatigue, helps improve visual acuity and depth perception, and increases blood flow to eye tissues.

- Brain health. Helps protect against aging and improves mental function.

- Sports-related activities. Promotes muscle endurance and protects against muscle damage.

- Diabetes, insulin resistance, and the metabolic syndrome. Helps improve antioxidant status and protects against vascular damage.

- Skin health. Reduces fine lines and wrinkles, improves skin elasticity, protects against sun damage, and prevents age spots and hyperpigmentation.

- Immune health. Protects against damage to immune cells.

Astaxanthin can cross the blood-brain and blood-retinal barriers to protect both the brain and eyes, an effect that is unusual for carotenes. Beta-carotene and lycopene do not cross either barrier. This effect of astaxanthin indicates that it may be particularly helpful in improving brain and eye health as well as protecting the brain against Alzheimer's disease, macular degeneration, and other degenerative brain and eye disorders. Of course, it has other benefits as well, but my thinking is that this ability to cross brain and retina barriers is what makes it special.

Although astaxanthin is found in salmon, herring roe, and krill oil supplements, the amounts in these sources are much lower than those provided from extracts of the microalga *Haematococcus pluvialis*. For example, the level of astaxanthin naturally occurring in a capsule of fish or krill oil is in the range of 100 mcg (0.1 mg). That amount is insignificant compared to the 3.5 mg per 4 ounces of sockeye salmon or the 4 to 12 mg per capsule found in most astaxanthin supplements derived from *H. pluvialis*.

Flavonoids

Flavonoids are a group of plant pigments that exert potent and effective antioxidant activity against a broader range of oxidants than the traditional antioxidants vitamins C and E, beta-carotene, selenium, and zinc. Besides lending color to fruits and flowers, flavonoids are responsible for many of the medicinal properties of foods, juices, herbs, and bee pollen. More than eight thousand flavonoid compounds have been classified according to their chemical structure. Flavonoids are sometimes called "nature's biological response modifiers" because of their anti-inflammatory, antiallergic, antiviral, and anticancer properties.

Recent research suggests that flavonoids may be useful in the support of many health conditions. In fact, many of the medicinal actions of foods, juices, herbs, and bee products such as pollen and propolis are now known to be directly related to their flavonoid content. Different flavonoids provide different benefits. For example, the flavonoids responsible for the red-to-blue colors of blueberries, blackberries, cherries, grapes, hawthorn berries, and many flowers are called anthocyanidins and proanthocyanidins. These flavonoids are found in the flesh of the fruit as well as the skin and possess an ability, among many others, to increase vitamin C levels within our cells, decrease the leakiness and breakage of small blood vessels, protect against free-radical damage, and support our joint structures.

Flavonoids also have a beneficial effect on collagen. Collagen, which is found in tendons, ligaments, and cartilage, is the most abundant protein in the body and is responsible for maintaining the integrity of "ground substance," which is responsible for holding the tissues of the body together.

The useful effects of flavonoids on collagen structures make them, especially those found in berries and cherries, helpful against arthritis and hardening of the arteries.

Flavonoids have the ability to protect the endothelial cells that line the blood vessels. Damage to these cells is what starts the process of atherosclerosis (hardening of the arteries) that ultimately leads to heart disease and strokes. Endothelial function also plays a role in inflammation, blood clotting, and blood flow. These benefits of flavonoids are especially important in protecting endothelial cells from the damaging effects of high blood sugar levels in people who have type 2 diabetes.

When researchers studied the diets of more than ten thousand men and women, they found that those who ate fruits and vegetables rich in various flavonoids had a lower risk of overall mortality and several chronic diseases, including heart disease, stroke, lung and prostate cancer, type 2 diabetes, and asthma.

Still other flavonoids are remarkable antiallergic compounds, modifying and reducing all phases of the allergic response. Specifically, they inhibit the formation and secretion of potent inflammatory compounds that produce the allergic response. Several prescription medications developed for allergic conditions (asthma, eczema, and hives) have been patterned after flavonoid molecules. An example of an antiallergy flavonoid is quercetin, which is available in many fruits and vegetables. Quercetin is an effective antioxidant that also inhibits the formation and release of histamine and other allergic compounds.

Due to their high flavonoid content, fruits and vegetables provide significant effects in improving a wide range of body functions. To get a sufficient dosage and to produce a synergetic effect, eat a variety of fruits and vegetables. Specific recommendations to achieve your flavonoid goal are discussed in chapter 6.

Types of Dietary Flavonoids		
Flavonoid Subclass	**Examples**	**Some Common Food Sources**
Anthocyanidins	Cyanidin, delphinidin, malvidin, pelargonidin, peonidin, petunidin	Red, blue, and purple berries; red and purple grapes; red wine; red cabbage
Flavanols	Monomers (catechins): catechin, epicatechin, epigallocatechin, epicatechin gallate, epigallocatechin gallate Dimers and polymers: theaflavins, thearubigins, proanthocyanidins	Catechins: teas (particularly green and white), chocolate, grapes, berries, apples Theaflavins, thearubigins: teas (particularly black and oolong) Proanthocyanidins: chocolate, apples, berries, grapes with seeds, red wine
Flavanones	Hesperetin, naringenin, eriodictyol	Citrus fruits, e.g., oranges, grapefruit, lemons
Flavonols	Quercetin, kaempferol, myricetin, isorhamnetin	Widely distributed: yellow onions, scallions, kale, broccoli, apples, berries, teas
Flavones	Apigenin, luteolin	Parsley, thyme, celery, cayenne pepper
Isoflavones	Daidzein, genistein, glycitein	Soybeans, soy foods, legumes

The Benefits of Eating a Rainbow of Fruits and Vegetables

Red: The Magic of Strawberries

The consumption of flavonoid sources such as strawberries, blueberries, apples, green tea, dark chocolate, and red wine has been shown in population studies to be associated with a significantly reduced risk for heart attacks and strokes. For example, data on 93,600 women from the Nurses' Health Study (NHS) II showed that a combined intake of greater than three servings per week of blueberries and strawberries was associated with a 34% decreased risk of having a heart attack compared to those who consumed the berries once a month or less.

The major benefits of strawberries and other flavonoid sources in protecting against cardiovascular disease is due largely to their effects on improving
the function of the endothelial cells that line the blood vessels. The endothelial
cells play a pivotal role in the regulation of vascular tone and structure as well
as vascular inflammation and clot formation. The lesions of atherosclerosis
(hardening of the arteries) first begin to develop with damage to endothelial
cells. Flavonoids, particularly the proanthocyanidin types found in berries, as
well as those found in other flavonoid-rich foods, have been shown to protect
and improve endothelial cell function.

In one study, healthy volunteers were supplemented daily with 500 grams
(about 2½ cups) of strawberries for one month. Strawberry consumption significantly reduced total cholesterol, low-density lipoprotein (LDL) cholesterol, and triglyceride levels (−8.78%, −13.72%, and −20.80%, respectively)
compared with the baseline period. Strawberry supplementation also significantly decreased various markers of oxidative stress. A significant increase
(>40%) in total plasma antioxidant capacity was also observed after strawberry
consumption. In addition, strawberry consumption improved platelet function, a key factor in preventing the formation of blood clots that can break off
and cause a heart attack, stroke, or pulmonary embolism.

Another study showed that even freeze-dried strawberries provided heart
health benefits. The study was designed to determine if freeze-dried strawberries (FDS) improved levels of blood lipids (cholesterol and triglycerides)
and lowered biomarkers of inflammation and lipid oxidation in adults with
abdominal obesity and elevated serum lipids. The sixty volunteers were
assigned to consume one of the following four beverages for twelve weeks: (1)
low-dose FDS (LD-FDS; 25 grams per day); (2) low-dose control (LD-C);
(3) high-dose FDS (HD-FDS; 50 grams per day); and (4) high-dose control
(HD-C). Control beverages were matched for calories, total fiber, appearance,
and taste. Results indicated a dose response to FDS as the high-dose group
experienced significantly greater decreases in serum total and LDL cholesterol compared to the group on the lower dosage.

Both doses of strawberries showed a similar decrease in a marker of antioxidant activity (serum malondialdehyde) at twelve weeks. In general, strawberry intervention did not affect blood pressure, blood sugar, serum concen-

trations of HDL cholesterol and triglycerides, or C-reactive protein (a marker of inflammation).

This study provides interesting results. Previous studies showed that higher fruit fiber intake had the greatest impact on reducing heart disease mortality, by as much as 32%. This study suggests that the benefit might be a combination of effects, including the lowering of cholesterol due to the fiber components. Even ingesting a reasonable amount of dried strawberries produces a clinically meaningful reduction in heart disease.

Red: The Magic of Tomatoes

Tomatoes contain lycopene, a red carotene also found in other red fruits and vegetables. Lycopene has received a lot of attention; it is protective against heart disease and the major cancers (breast, colon, lung, skin, and prostate). In one of the more detailed studies of lycopene, Harvard University researchers discovered that men who consumed the highest levels of lycopene (6.5 mg per day) showed a 21% decreased risk of prostate cancer compared with those consuming the lowest levels. Men who ate two or more servings of tomato sauce each week were 23% less likely to develop prostate cancer during the twenty-two-year study than men who ate less than one serving of tomato sauce each month. Lycopene consumption has also been shown to lower the risk of heart disease, cataracts, and macular degeneration. Population-based studies have shown that consumption of more than seven servings per week of tomato-based products is associated with a 30% reduction in the risk of heart disease.

Many of the benefits of tomatoes and lycopene are thought to be due to their ability to fight inflammation, especially in obesity. In obesity, the increased level of body fat leads to an increase in circulating inflammatory mediators. Since lycopene has been shown to reduce markers of inflammation, researchers have hypothesized that the consumption of tomatoes and other lycopene-rich foods may help to reduce inflammation in people who are overweight or obese.

Drinking a glass of tomato juice daily may produce anti-inflammatory benefits. In one double-blind study, groups of overweight and obese women were given either 330 ml per day of tomato juice or water for twenty days.

At baseline and day 20, serum concentrations of inflammatory mediators were compared. The results showed that tomato juice reduced the presence of important compounds linked to inflammation. It is thought that frequent consumption of tomatoes may help to reduce the risk of developing chronic diseases linked to inflammation, such as heart disease, cancer, and diabetes.

The absorption of lycopene is highly dependent on the tomato product being consumed. The redder the tomato, the higher the lycopene content. The more the tomato is processed, the better the lycopene is absorbed by the body, because processing liberates more lycopene from the plant's cells. The absorption of lycopene from tomato paste, sauce, or juice is five times as great as that from raw tomatoes. Consuming a lycopene source together with extra-virgin olive oil can also improve its absorption.

To determine the effect of typical servings of commercially available tomato products on blood and prostate lycopene concentrations, researchers at Ohio State University assigned men scheduled to undergo removal of their prostate glands due to cancer to either a lycopene-restricted control group (<5 mg lycopene per day) or to groups providing 25 to 35 mg of lycopene per day from the following tomato products: tomato soup (2 to 2¾ cups per day); tomato sauce (5 to 7 ounces per day); or vegetable juice (11 to 16.5 fluid ounces per day).

Tomato soup, sauce, and juice consumption significantly increased plasma lycopene concentration by 66%, 71%, and 59%, respectively, while the controls consuming the lycopene-restricted diet showed a decline in plasma lycopene concentration by 24%. The end-of-study prostate lycopene concentration was 3.5-, 3.6-, and 2.2-fold higher in the tomato soup, sauce, and juice consumers, respectively.

Interestingly, in the tomato products, 80% to 90% of the lycopene was in the trans (linear) configuration, while in the blood and prostate isomers 47% and 80%, respectively, were in the cis (bent) form. This difference demonstrates a shift toward cis accumulation and perhaps a preference for the cis isomer over the trans in the prostate and other body tissues.

Previous studies have shown that the cis form is also better absorbed—55% greater than the trans form. You can increase the cis form by heating tomato paste at 260°F for at least forty minutes. Heating or cooking the tomato paste will increase the amount of cis isomers ninefold. Be sure to add 1 tablespoon extra-virgin olive oil to further increase absorption. When lycopene is in its trans, or linear, form it tends to stack and become crystallized, which lowers, but does not eliminate, its absorption. In the cis form, lycopene is able to mix more easily with the olive oil and be transported into the blood.

My recommendation is to consume 10 mg of lycopene every day. I get my 10 mg of lycopene in supplemental form. Why take a lycopene pill? Because I don't eat enough tomato sauce or paste on a daily basis.

Red: The Magic of Cherries

One of the most popular medicinal uses of cherries, cherry juice, and cherry extracts has been the treatment and prevention of gout. Gout is a painful form of arthritis characterized by increased blood levels of uric acid and the formation of uric acid crystals in joints. Cherries, like many other berries, are rich sources of anthocyanidins and proanthocyanidins. These compounds are flavonoid molecules that are remarkable in their ability to prevent destruction to connective tissue and joints.

Consuming the equivalent of 8 ounces of fresh cherries per day was shown in a 1950 study to be effective in lowering uric acid levels and preventing attacks of gout. Since then additional studies have confirmed these benefits:

- Results from a study in healthy women who ate a bowl of Bing cherries for breakfast indicated that the cherry intake lowered blood levels of uric acid. Eating cherries also increased the urinary excretion of uric acid and lowered markers of inflammation such as C-reactive protein (a chemical produced by the liver that increases rapidly during inflammation, such as during a gout attack) and nitric oxide (a chemical that is also involved in damaging arthritic joints).

- In a follow-up study, healthy men and women who consumed the equivalent of 45 cherries per day for twenty-eight days showed a significant reduction in C-reactive protein and nitric oxide.

In the most recent study, conducted by researchers from the Boston University School of Medicine, cherry intake was again shown to reduce gout attacks. The study recruited 633 people with gout and followed them online for a year. Participants answered questions about gout onset, symptoms, risk factors, medications, and whether they ate cherries or took cherry extract, and for how long.

When the researchers analyzed the participants' responses, they found that cherry intake (defined as ½ cup or 10 to 12 cherries or the equivalent in extract form) over a two-day period was associated with a 35% lower risk of gout attacks and that cherry extract intake was associated with a 45% lower risk. The risk of gout attacks was reduced by 75% when cherry intake was combined with allopurinol, the standard drug used to treat gout. These benefits persisted even after other factors that can affect gout risk, such as gender, obesity, and purine intake (which can increase gout risk), plus the use of alcohol, diuretics, and antigout medications, were considered.

Fresh cherries are available from late spring through summer in various areas of North America. Frozen cherries can be used throughout the year in smoothies and juices.

Red: The Magic of Watermelon

While medicine has focused primarily on watermelon's diuretic effects, research indicates that drinking watermelon juice is a postworkout remedy that can help reduce muscle soreness.

Watermelon is an excellent source of the amino acid citrulline, which the human body converts to arginine and nitric oxide, a key regulator of blood flow. Available as a dietary supplement, citrulline is showing benefits in treating Alzheimer's disease, dementia, fatigue, muscle weakness, erectile dysfunction, high blood pressure, and diabetes. Many of these effects are also achieved with arginine supplementation. The advantage of citrulline over arginine is that it provides a more prolonged boost in blood arginine levels. The same may be true of watermelon juice.

In a small study conducted at a Spanish university, researchers monitored seven athletes after they exerted maximum effort on a stationary bike. On different days, the athletes were supplied with 500 ml of natural watermelon juice (1.17 grams of citrulline), enriched watermelon juice (4.83 grams of citrulline plus 1.17 grams from watermelon), or a placebo. Results showed that both of the watermelon juices helped to reduce the recovery heart rate and muscle soreness after twenty-four hours compared to the placebo.

The study seems to indicate that the citrulline from watermelon may be better absorbed or utilized than that from a supplement. In another part of the study, the researchers used a laboratory model to compare the absorption of citrulline from unpasteurized or pasteurized watermelon juice compared to citrulline as a supplement. The result showed that the bioavailability of citrulline was greater in the raw juice than either the pasteurized juice or the solution containing citrulline. These results show the advantage of drinking fresh fruit and vegetable juices.

Watermelon is cooling and refreshing. Eat pieces of watermelon or juice it with other ingredients.

Orange: The Magic of Mangoes

More mangoes are consumed throughout the world than apples or any other fruit. Mangoes come in more than a thousand varieties. They range in shape and size from round to kidney-shaped and from diminutive plum size to melon-size fruits weighing up to four pounds. Most commercially grown varieties are about the size and shape of a large avocado. One exception is the Manila mango, a pear-size, golden-yellow variety beginning to appear in US markets.

Mangoes have high concentrations of carotenoids, antioxidant nutrients, and various phytochemicals. Research conducted in 2002 by Dr. Sue Percival, an associate professor with the University of Florida's Institute of Food and Agricultural Sciences, showed that mangoes can inhibit the formation and growth of cancer cells. Interestingly, Percival compared an organic extract containing mango's carotenes to a water-soluble mango extract in their effectiveness against cancer formation. According to her findings, mango's water-soluble portion was about ten times more effective in preventing cancer cell formation than its carotenes. Compounds in the aqueous portion of the mango include not only water-soluble nutrients such as vitamin C, but also valuable flavonoid compounds.

Human evidence also demonstrates that mangoes can help fight cancer. A diet analysis of 64 patients with gallbladder cancer and 101 patients with gallstones showed that mango consumption was correlated with a 60% reduction in risk for gallbladder cancer—the highest reduction in risk for this cancer found for any fruit or vegetable.

The mango may also offer some protection against infections. The Department of Epidemiology and International Health at the University of Alabama conducted a four-month study of 176 Gambian children. Those who received dried mango were found to have higher blood levels of retinol (vitamin A) than those who were given a placebo. Since vitamin A's nickname is "the anti-infective vitamin," the mango may literally be a lifesaving fruit in developing countries where there can be a severe seasonal shortage of carotenoid-rich foods. In other studies indicating the mango's protective effects on overall health, infants in Gambia and India were found to have the best gut integrity and thus the least intestinal disease and diarrhea during the three-month period when mangoes were in season in each country.

In a Mexican study, eating mango was shown to afford protection against giardia, an organism responsible for what is often referred to as "traveler's diarrhea." In people who developed traveler's diarrhea due to giardia, consuming mango was found to eliminate the giardia just as well as tinidazole, a drug commonly used to treat giardia infection.

Yellow: The Magic of Lemons

Lemons, especially their peels, are an excellent source of molecules known as terpenes, such as d-limonene. Naturally occurring terpenes are used as alternatives to synthetic terpenes in many natural cleaning products. The primary health benefits of terpenes revolve around some impressive anticancer effects—both in prevention and possibly in treatment. For example, six individuals with advanced cancers were able to halt the progression of their cancer for periods of time ranging from six to twelve months while taking d-limonene.

In a study conducted at the University of Arizona Cancer Center, forty-three women with newly diagnosed operable breast cancer who elected to undergo lumpectomy (surgical excision) were given 2 grams of d-limonene daily for two to six weeks before surgery. Blood and breast tissue were collected to determine the level of d-limonene and its metabolites as well as changes in systemic and tissue biomarkers of breast cancer risk or carcinogenesis. Results showed that d-limonene concentrated preferentially in the breast tissue, reaching a high tissue concentration (average = 41.3 µg per g tissue), whereas the major active circulating metabolite, perillic acid, did not concentrate in the breast tissue.

Results also showed that d-limonene supplementation resulted in a 22% reduction in the expression of tumor markers. Specifically, d-limonene reduced the expression of breast tumor cyclin D1. Cyclin D1 is one of the frequently overexpressed proteins and one of the commonly amplified genes in breast cancer. The gene that leads to cyclin D1 formation is an estrogen-responsive gene. The overexpression of cyclin D1 occurs in more than half of invasive breast cancers. Recent evidence also shows that cyclin D1 interferes with the anticancer effect of tamoxifen in estrogen receptor–positive breast cancers, potentially accounting for treatment failure with tamoxifen therapy. For obvious reasons, the benefits seen with d-limonene in this study should be followed up in women with breast cancer who are expressing cyclin D1.

Given the safety and potential benefit of d-limonene, eating more lemons makes sense in the battle against breast cancer. The highest content of d-limonene is found in the lemon peel and white spongy inner parts. A typical average-size lemon has about 300 mg of d-limonene.

The best way to take advantage of lemons' health benefits is to drink the juice. Since lemon juice is too tart on its own, mix it with other juices or make lemonade by mixing it with sparkling mineral water and stevia or another zero- or low-calorie natural sweetener. I also recommend adding a half or one whole lemon (complete with peel) to just about any fresh fruit or green vegetable juice.

Whenever possible, choose organic lemons over conventionally grown ones. If you can't find organic lemons, soak or spray conventionally grown ones with a biodegradable wash, then rinse well.

Other dietary sources of terpenes are other citrus fruits, berries, cherries, and volatile herbs such as peppermint, basil, thyme, and rosemary.

Green: The Magic of Kale

One serving of kale has more calcium than a glass of milk. Kale and other dark leafy greens are packed with vitamin K_1, which helps convert a bone protein known as osteocalcin, a major noncollagen protein, into an active form. Osteocalcin's role is to anchor calcium molecules and hold them in place within the bone.

A deficiency of vitamin K leads to impaired mineralization of the bone due to inadequate osteocalcin levels. Very low blood levels of vitamin K_1 have been found in patients with fractures due to osteoporosis. The severity of fracture is strongly correlated with the level of circulating vitamin K: the lower the level of vitamin K, the more severe the fracture. Green leafy vegetables are the best source of vitamin K, making them ideal for omnivores, vegetarians, and vegans in the fight against osteoporosis.

In addition to calcium and vitamin K_1, the high levels of many trace minerals in green leafy vegetables may be responsible for this protective effect. Boron is a trace mineral that is gaining attention as a protective factor against osteoporosis. It has been shown to have a positive effect on calcium and active estrogen levels in postmenopausal women, the group at highest risk for developing osteoporosis. In one study, supplementing the diet of postmenopausal women with 3 mg of boron per day reduced urinary calcium excretion by 44% and dramatically increased the levels of the most biologically active estrogen. Boron is required to activate certain hormones involved in bone health, including estrogen and vitamin D. Since fruits and vegetables are the main dietary sources of boron, diets low in these foods may be deficient in boron.

Green: The Magic of Broccoli

Broccoli and other members of the cabbage family demonstrate remarkable anticancer effects, particularly in breast cancer. Compounds known as glucosinolates in cabbage-family vegetables such as broccoli, kale, and brussels sprouts increase the excretion of the form of estrogen (2-hydroxyestrone) linked to breast cancer.

One of the key isothiocyanates in broccoli is sulforaphane. This compound was first identified in broccoli sprouts grown in plastic laboratory dishes by scientists at the Johns Hopkins University School of Medicine in Baltimore, Maryland. The researchers were investigating the anticancer compounds present in broccoli when they discovered that broccoli sprouts contain anywhere from thirty to fifty times the concentration of protective chemicals found in mature broccoli plants. Feeding sulforophane-rich broccoli sprout extracts dramatically reduced the frequency, size, and number of tumors in laboratory rats exposed to a standard carcinogen. Human studies with sulforaphane have shown that these compounds stimulate the body's production of detoxification enzymes and exert antioxidant effects.

A study published in *Proceedings of the National Academy of Sciences* has shown that sulforaphane may be quite helpful in improving symptoms of autism. Nearly half of forty males aged 13 to 27 with moderate to severe autism spectrum disorder (ASD) showed significant improvement after taking sulforaphane at a daily dose of 50 to 150 µmol for eighteen weeks. Significantly greater improvement was shown among participants in the treatment group at four, ten, and eighteen weeks for irritability, lethargy, and hyperactivity as well as awareness, communication, motivation, and mannerism. At eighteen weeks, 46% of the treatment group was much improved in social interaction, aberrant behavior, and verbal communication, compared to 0% for those in the placebo group. After discontinuation of sulforaphane treatment, all scales reverted back to the baseline levels.

Autism is associated with poor antioxidant protection and an impaired ability to detoxify harmful chemicals. This combination creates inflammation within cells leading to dysfunction of the mitochondria, the energy-producing compartments of the cell. The end result is that the nerve cells in the brain do not function properly. Sulforaphane increases the ability of the cell's antioxidant, detoxification, and anti-inflammatory system to quench the fire and restore more optimal function. It does this by a combination of effects, including stimulating expression of the genes that fight these aberrations as well as exerting some direct actions on its own. Basically, the same mechanisms that make cabbage-family vegetables so beneficial in fighting cancer may also be important in improving autism.

Green: The Magic of Spinach

Many greens, especially spinach, are high sources of lutein, a yellow-orange carotene that appears to provide significant protection against age-related macular degeneration (ARMD). The macula is the area of the retina where images are focused; it is the portion of the eye responsible for fine vision. Degeneration of the macula is the leading cause of severe visual loss in the United States. The macula, especially the central portion of the macula (the fovea) owes its yellow color to its high concentration of lutein.

A low level of lutein in the macula is a major risk factor for ARMD. Therefore, increasing the concentration of lutein within the macula provides significant protective effects against the development of macular degeneration. Increasing the lutein content of the diet as well as supplementing with lutein has been shown to increase blood and macular lutein concentrations, a worthwhile goal in both the prevention and treatment of macular degeneration.

In addition to carotenes such as lutein, researchers have identified at least thirteen different flavonoid compounds in spinach that function as antioxidants and anticancer agents. The anticancer properties of spinach flavonoids have been sufficiently impressive to prompt researchers to create specialized spinach extracts to be used in controlled studies. These extracts have been shown to slow down cell division in stomach cancer cells (gastric adenocarcinomas) and, in studies on mice, to reduce skin cancers (skin papillomas). A study of adult women living in New England in the late 1980s also showed intake of spinach to be inversely related to incidence of breast cancer. Though the study was done a long time ago, the results are quite significant.

The key point is that even though a plant may be one color and provide significant levels of a particular pigment, remember that there are other compounds, including other pigments, that exert additional health benefits.

Blue: The Magic of Blueberries

These nutritional power packets are rich in plant pigments known as anthocyanidins, a type of flavonoid that is responsible for the berries' dark blue-purple color. When researchers at Tufts University analyzed sixty fruits and vegetables for their antioxidant capability, blueberries came out on top, rating highest in their capacity to destroy free radicals. Their anthocyanidin content is the reason why.

While blueberries have long been used for a wide range of medicinal effects, it is their ability to improve vision that is now the most popular medicinal application. This use was stimulated by the fact that during World War II, British Royal Air Force pilots consumed bilberry (a variety of European blueberry) preserves before their night missions. The pilots believed, based on folk medicine, that the bilberries would improve their ability to see at night. After the war, numerous studies demonstrated that blueberry extracts do in fact improve nighttime visual acuity and lead to quicker adjustment to darkness and faster restoration of visual acuity after exposure to glare. Clinical studies have shown good results in individuals with sensitivity to bright lights, diabetic retinopathy, and macular degeneration. Additional research points out that bilberries may be protective against the development of cataracts and glaucoma and quite therapeutic in the treatment of varicose veins, hemorrhoids, and peptic ulcers.

Blueberries are also important in preserving brain function as we age. In animal studies, researchers found that blueberries help protect the brain from oxidative stress and may reduce the effects of age-related conditions such as Alzheimer's disease and dementia. Researchers found that feeding rats the human equivalent of a cup of blueberries a day significantly improved both the learning capacity and motor skills of aging rats, making them mentally equivalent to much younger rats. Not only did the rats given the blueberries learn faster than those in the other group, but their motor skills also improved. When the rats' brains were examined, the brain cells of the ones given blueberries were found to communicate more effectively than those of the others.

Blueberries also promote urinary tract health. They contain the same compounds found in cranberries that help prevent or eliminate urinary tract infections. In order for bacteria to cause an infection, they must first adhere to the mucosal lining of the urethra and bladder. Components found in cranberry and blueberry juice block the ability of bacteria such as E. coli to adhere to the lining of the bladder. Since the bacteria can't adhere to the bladder lining, they are washed away during urination.

Flavonoid sources such as berries, apples, green tea, dark chocolate, and red wine have all been shown in population studies to be associated with a significantly reduced risk of heart attacks and strokes. Data on 93,600 women from the Nurses' Health Study (NHS) II showed that a combined intake of more than three servings a week of blueberries and strawberries was associated with a 34% decreased risk of having a heart attack compared to those consuming berries once a month or less.

In a study conducted at Florida State University, blueberry consumption lowered blood pressure. Forty-eight postmenopausal women with mild hypertension were enrolled to evaluate the effects of daily blueberry consumption for eight weeks. The women were randomly assigned to receive either 22 grams of freeze-dried blueberry powder or 22 grams of control powder daily. Approximately 22 grams of freeze-dried blueberry powder is equal to one cup of fresh blueberries, an attainable dosage for people to consume on a daily basis. After eight weeks, the subjects ingesting the blueberry powder had an average lower blood pressure (131/75 mm Hg) compared to their average baseline level (138/80 mm Hg), whereas there were no changes in the group receiving the control powder. Blueberry consumption was also associated with improved arterial flexibility.

The biggest change, however, was in the subjects' nitric oxide levels. Nitric oxide plays a central role in determining the tone of blood vessels. Specifically, it exerts a relaxing effect on them, thereby increasing blood flow. It also improves blood fluidity and reduces blood clot formation. Results showed that the average nitric oxide level of the subjects taking the blueberry powder was greater (15.35 μmol/L) at eight weeks compared with their average baseline value (9.11 μmol/L), whereas there were no changes in the control group.

These results show that daily blueberry consumption may reduce blood pressure and, perhaps more important, improve arterial stiffness the same way as beets (see page 93).

See Berries under "My 7 Favorite Superfoods" (page 98) for more information.

Purple: The Magic of Beets

More than sixty million Americans have high blood pressure, including more than half (54.3%) of all Americans 65 to 74 years old and almost three-quarters (71.8%) of all American blacks in the same age group. High blood pressure is a major risk factor for a heart attack or stroke. In fact, it is regarded as the most significant risk factor for a stroke.

Recently, there have been several studies showing that drinking fresh beet juice can lead to clinically meaningful reductions in blood pressure. Beet juice has been a popular folk remedy for centuries. The primary focus has been in disorders of the liver, but beet juice has recently gained recognition for its anticancer and heart health–promoting properties.

The pigment that gives beets their rich purple-crimson color—betacyanin—is a powerful cancer-fighting agent, while naturally occurring nitrates in the beets are thought to be responsible for their beneficial effects on the heart and vascular system. Studies with beet juice have shown that:

- Drinking just 16 ounces of fresh beet juice a day significantly reduced blood pressure by up to 10 mm Hg in healthy subjects.

- After drinking 16 ounces of beet juice, blood pressure was lower within just an hour, with the peak drop occurring three to four hours after ingestion. The decrease in blood pressure is due to the chemical formation of nitrite from the nitrates in the juice.

- Once in the general circulation, nitrite can be converted to nitric oxide by the cells that line blood vessels. Nitric oxide is a powerful dilator of blood vessels, resulting in lower blood pressure. Drinking beet juice is considerably more effective in raising blood nitrite levels than eating an equivalent amount of nitrate-rich foods.

In one of the most detailed studies on beet juice, researchers at the Baker Heart and Diabetes Institute in Melbourne, Australia, had fifteen men and fifteen women drink either 17.6 ounces of a beet juice beverage containing

500 grams of beet and apple juice (72% beet, 28% apple) or a placebo. The participants' blood pressure was measured at baseline and at least hourly for twenty-four hours following juice consumption using an ambulatory blood pressure monitor. The same procedure was repeated two weeks later, with those who drank the placebo in the first round drinking beet juice in the second and vice versa. Those who drank beet juice had a systolic blood pressure an average of four to five points lower after six hours. The significance of this is that drinking beet juice could cut the rate of strokes and heart attacks by about 10%. In terms of lives, that would mean about sixty thousand lives saved each year in the United States.

These are just some of the many thousands of beneficial fruits and vegetables; eating a variety of them will produce the greatest synergetic effect on your health and well-being. When you're hungry, reach for fruits and vegetables; they contain the true magic of food.

6

My Favorite Superfoods

My definition of a superfood is one that provides exceptional health benefits. My list of superfoods is somewhat different from most because my general diet recommendations focus on already popular superfoods, such as berries, fatty fish, legumes, whole grains, and dark leafy greens.

When it comes to superfoods, many people suffer from xenophilia. *Xeno* means "foreign," and *philia* means "love." We tend to think of exotic, foreign-sounding fruits and vegetables as being better than the common fruits and vegetables that are readily available. Apples, cranberries, and grapes are just as good for you and less expensive than exotic acai, goji berries, and mangosteens.

Before explaining the superfoods I've included, it's important to understand some of the basic science about why they are so important and what to look for.

Superfoods and Flavonoids

To eat a diet rich in antioxidant activity, you should focus on flavonoids, a type of plant pigment and a member of the larger polyphenol family. As a class of compounds, the more than eight thousand flavonoids are sometimes called "nature's biological response modifiers" because of their anti-inflammatory, antiallergic, antiviral, and anticancer properties. Many superfoods owe their benefits to their flavonoid content. Though different flavonoids have different effects in the body, the key factor may not be a high intake of any one particular flavonoid but rather a high total flavonoid intake that also provides a high variety of flavonoids rather than any one particular flavonoid class.

Research shows that it does not seem to matter where the flavonoids come from, e.g., through dietary sources, such as legumes, fruits, green tea, coffee, chocolate, or through flavonoid-rich extracts, such as ginkgo, milk thistle, or bilberry, as long as an effective dosage is being taken. The caveat is that the proanthocyanidin flavonoids must be a major part of the flavonoid intake. Good dietary sources of these compounds are found in red or black grapes (especially the seeds), apples, cacao, cocoa, dark chocolate, berries (especially blueberries, cranberries, and black currants), certain nuts (especially hazelnuts, pecans, and pistachios), and red wine.

Keeping this caveat on the importance of proanthocyanidins in mind, what is an effective dosage of flavonoids? Let's take a look at that question by applying concepts in pharmacology, or how a drug works. One of the key terms in pharmacology is *effective dose*, which means the dose or amount of drug that produces a therapeutic response or desired effect in some fraction of the subjects taking it. For example, the ED50 is the effective dose for 50% of people receiving the drug. Another way of looking at ED50 is that half of the people taking the drug would not notice an effect. The ED95 is the dose required to achieve a desired effect in 95% of people taking the drug.

With drugs, there is usually a clear effect being looked for in a relatively short period of time. With diet, the effects can be immediate in some cases, but in the prevention of such things as heart disease and cancer, it is much more difficult to determine the effect because these diseases take so long to develop. That is where large population-based (epidemiological) studies can provide valuable clues. Based upon population-based studies as well as some of the clinical assessments, there appears to be a threshold for observing many of the key beneficial effects of flavonoid intake. Looking at the population-based studies with green tea is an example of the importance of trying to quantify how much of a particular food was consumed. Studies on green tea in preventing cancer or heart disease are often interpreted as showing mixed results.

However, if we look at the studies that properly determined the amount of green tea polyphenols that were consumed, there is a clear benefit and a definite dose effect.

The best evidence for determining the effective dosage of total flavonoid intake is from clinical trials with well-defined sources of flavonoids either from foods and beverages or from flavonoid-rich extracts. Fortunately, there has been an explosion of good scientific studies on a wide variety of flavonoid sources. They have focused on proanthocyanidin-rich extracts of cocoa, grape seed, and pine bark, as well as flavonoid-rich extracts of pomegranate, citrus, soy, and green tea. Some of these studies have shown significant clinical benefits in the following health conditions: asthma; atherosclerosis (hardening of the arteries); attention deficit disorder; high blood pressure; high cholesterol levels; male infertility; mild cognitive impairment; menopausal symptoms; osteoarthritis; periodontal disease; varicose veins, venous insufficiency, and capillary fragility; and visual function, retinopathy, and macular degeneration.

There have also been a large number of studies of flavonoid-rich sources looking at more immediate effects, such as their effect on blood vessel function, blood flow, or antioxidant capacity. Most of the studies with the aforementioned flavonoid-rich extracts have used an average dosage of about 300 mg per day to show an effect. The same is true for the dosage of most herbal sources of flavonoids, such as ginkgo, hawthorn berry, and milk thistle extract. To determine the effective total flavonoid intake, we can look at all of the evidence from population-based studies, clinical trials in certain health conditions, and the effects noted in clinical trials evaluating a specific body function.

Based upon my interpretation of all of these data, I believe that the total flavonoid intake to achieve an ED95 is at least 500 mg daily from a wide variety of sources. The Synergetic Diet is high in flavonoid content because of its dietary and supplementation strategy, so you don't have to do the measuring. For many years, I have personally tried to consume a minimum of 2,000 mg of flavonoids per day and on most days go well beyond this number. Remember, these foods also contain numerous other beneficial compounds. Here is a list of the high-flavonoid foods and supplements that I consume on a daily basis to reach this goal.

Dr. Murray's Daily Intake of Flavonoids		
	Daily Dosage	Flavonoid Content
Dietary Sources		
Berries	1 cup	205 mg
Raw cacao powder	3 tablespoons	85 mg
Tea (green or herbal)	12 ounces	400 mg
Nuts	⅓ to ½ cup	35 mg
General diet not included above	—	150 mg
Supplement Sources		
Micronized diosmin	600 mg	600 mg
Resveratrol	500 mg	500 mg
Cacao flavonols	375 mg	375 mg
Grape seed extract	300 mg	300 mg
Green Tea Phytosome	300 mg	100 mg

My 7 Favorite Superfoods

Though there is little doubt that many common fruits, vegetables, legumes, nuts, seeds, spices, herbs, and other foods are worthy of superfood status, here are the ones that I eat and drink on a daily basis because of their exceptional health properties.

1. Berries

Though I said that my list of superfoods is different from others', I start with a superfood on everyone's list: berries. Though some lists focus on one type of berry, I encourage you to eat a variety of them, including blackberries, blueberries, raspberries, strawberries, cranberries, currants, acai, gojis, and others. Berries are rich in vital nutrients and phytochemicals such as flavonoids, yet low in calories, making them an excellent food choice if you have a sweet tooth and are attempting to improve the nutritional quality of the foods you eat without increasing the number of calories consumed.

Most of the research on the beneficial effects of berries has focused on blueberries, cranberries, black currants, and strawberries; other top fruit sources include pomegranate, amla (gooseberry), grapes (with seeds), and cherries.

Though I have stressed the importance of flavonoids, berries also contain many other beneficial phytochemicals. Whereas blueberries, for example, are higher in anthocyanidin flavonoids, strawberries are a much better source of the anticancer compound ellagic acid. In one study, strawberries topped a list of eight foods most linked to lower rates of cancer deaths among a group of 1,271 elderly people in New Jersey. Those eating the most strawberries were one-third as likely to develop cancer as those eating fewer or no strawberries. Again, the key is to eat a variety of berries daily to make sure you are getting an array of flavonoids and other beneficial compounds that act synergistically.

Try to eat at least one cup of mixed berries every day.

2. Raw Cacao Powder and Dark Chocolate

Cacao and cocoa both come from the beans of the cacao tree, but raw cacao beans are minimally processed to produce raw cacao powder by crushing the beans to remove the fat. The result is a powder that looks similar to cocoa powder, but the latter is roasted and, in the process, loses many of its key compounds and living enzymes.

Of all the foods available on planet Earth, perhaps the most magical and best loved are those from cacao, especially chocolate. Chocolate is produced from the beans of the cacao tree, whose scientific name, *Theobroma cacao*, reflects our long-standing love of chocolate (*theobroma* being Greek for "food of the gods").

Including some chocolate in your diet has many health benefits. At the center of these are the flavonoids contained in chocolate. While these plant pigments are responsible for many of the health benefits of numerous fruits and medicinal plants, chocolate delivers them in a much more sensually pleasing way. Also, there is evidence that not only is chocolate rich in flavonoids, but factors in chocolate somehow dramatically increase the absorption of these compounds. The key flavonoids are flavonols similar to those found in green tea, as well as proanthocyanidins (also called procyanidins), similar to those found in grape seed extracts, berries, and pine bark extract. Chocolate is replete with both of these compounds. In fact, flavonoids constitute as much as 48% of the dry weight of the cocoa bean. Cocoa powder can contain as much as 10% flavonoids on a dry-weight basis, with dark chocolate being the best source.

One of the key areas of research into the benefits of chocolate consumption is its effect on cardiovascular disease. A growing amount of research suggests that chocolate is a rich source of flavonoid antioxidants that are especially important in protecting against damage to "good" cholesterol and the lining of the arteries. Chocolate flavonoids prevent the excessive clumping together of blood platelets that can cause blood clots. Unlike the saturated fats found in meat and dairy products, the saturated fats found in chocolate do not elevate cholesterol levels. Cocoa butter contains small amounts of the plant sterols sitosterol and stigmasterol, which may help inhibit the absorption of dietary cholesterol. Chocolate, like nuts, provides significant amounts of arginine, an amino acid that is required in the production of nitric oxide. Nitric oxide helps regulate blood flow, inflammation, and blood pressure.

In order to show how chocolate improves cardiovascular health, a more detailed anatomy lesson is required. As described in the previous chapter, all blood vessels, from the heart to the smallest capillary, have an endothelial cell lining, or endothelium. If all of the endothelial cells in the body were laid out flat, the endothelial surface area would be about the size of a football field. It is the effect of chocolate polyphenols on endothelial cells that ultimately is responsible for the most important health benefits of chocolate.

The loss of proper endothelial function is a hallmark of vascular diseases and is often regarded as a key early event in the development of atherosclerosis (hardening of the arteries). Impaired endothelial function is often seen in patients with diabetes, hypertension, and high cholesterol levels, as well as in smokers.

The main causes of endothelial dysfunction are high blood sugar levels and damage caused by free radicals and pro-oxidants. One of the key consequences of this damage is a diminished ability to manufacture nitric oxide. The importance of this chemical messenger used by the endothelial cells was discussed previously in explaining how beets lower blood pressure.

Cocoa Improves Brain Function

One of the major contributors to impaired mental function as we age is reduced blood flow to the brain. Natural approaches designed to improve blood flow to the brain show significant promise in the prevention and treatment of mild cognitive impairment. A 2013 study conducted by Harvard University researchers shows that drinking hot cocoa is beneficial.

To investigate the relationship between cocoa consumption and brain health, a group of sixty people (aged 72.9 ± 5.4 years) without dementia was studied in a double-blind clinical trial. The participants drank two cups of hot cocoa per day for thirty days and did not consume any other chocolate during the study. One group consumed a high-flavonol hot cocoa providing 609 mg of cocoa flavonols; the other group consumed a low-flavonol version providing 13 mg.

At the beginning of the study and then again after thirty days, the participants were given tests of memory and thinking skills and ultrasound tests to measure the amount of blood flow to the brain during the tests.

What these researchers and others showed is that as different areas of the brain need more energy to complete their tasks, they also need greater blood flow. This relationship, called neurovascular coupling, plays a role in development of dementia and/or Alzheimer's disease.

Of the sixty participants, eighteen had impaired blood flow at the start of the study. Those people had an 8.3% improvement in blood flow to the working areas of the brain by the end of the study, while there was no improvement for those who started out with regular blood flow.

Those with impaired blood flow also improved their times on a test of working memory, with scores dropping from 167 seconds at the beginning of the study to 116 seconds at the end. There was no change in times for people with regular blood flow. A total of twenty-four of the participants also had MRI scans of the brain to look for tiny areas of brain damage. The scans found that people with impaired blood flow were also more likely to have such areas.

Interestingly, there was no clear difference between the two study groups. In other words, both the high- and low-flavonol hot cocoas were shown to produce benefits. This outcome suggests that flavonol molecules are not the only beneficial compounds in chocolate and hot cocoa. Other beneficial compounds that could have contributed to the effects noted include theobromine (a caffeinelike compound) and arginine, an amino acid that is required in the production of nitric oxide. Nitric oxide helps regulate blood flow, inflammation, and blood pressure.

How Much Chocolate to Eat

To make the healthiest chocolate choices, let me offer some suggestions. For the biggest flavonoid bang for your caloric buck, always choose high-quality dark chocolate. Read the label: the cocoa content should be 70% or more. The higher the cocoa content beyond 70%, the more bitter the chocolate will taste. I personally like 85% cocoa content, but some people find it way too bitter.

There are a lot of good choices out there for delicious healthful chocolate sources. My favorite bars are from Good Superfoods (www.goodsuperfoods .com). There are other great brands out there, but try to purchase organic, fair-trade chocolate.

Most experts agree that the recommended daily "dose" is 1 to 2 ounces dark chocolate. To help meter your chocolate intake, consider buying dark chocolate bars in small serving sizes such as 0.35-ounce bites. Several brands, including Ghirardelli and Lindt, as well as health food store brands such as Endangered Species, offer dark chocolate bites. Enjoy one as an after-meal treat.

I get my cacao fix from a special brew that I make almost every day with organic raw cacao powder. For a hot beverage, stir 2 to 3 tablespoons raw cacao powder, 1 tablespoon xylitol or erythritol, and 1 teaspoon stevia into a large mug. Fill the mug with brewed coffee (I use decaf). You can also stir in one of the following: ½ to 1 teaspoon ground cinnamon, 1 drop pure vanilla extract, a dash of grated nutmeg, or a drop of peppermint oil.

3. Green Tea

The world's most popular teas come from *Camellia sinensis*, the source of both green and black teas. Four times as much black tea is produced and consumed as green tea. Though black tea is more popular, green tea provides greater health benefits.

The difference between green and black teas results from the manufacturing process. To produce black tea, the leaves are allowed to oxidize. A series of chemical reactions is allowed to take place that result in the browning of the tea leaves and the production of flavor and aroma compounds. Unfortunately, during oxidation, enzymes present in the tea convert the polyphenols into substances with much less biological activity. In contrast, green tea is produced by lightly steaming the fresh-cut leaf. Steaming prevents the enzymes from converting the polyphenols, so oxidation does not take place. Oolong tea is partially oxidized.

White tea is still green tea, but the new, unopened buds are steamed or dried after picking. The resulting tea is pale yellow and low in caffeine and tastes mild and slightly sweeter than green tea.

The Magic of Green Tea

Although green tea contains vitamins and minerals, the polyphenols are the primary keys to its magic. The usual concentration of total polyphenols, a larger category of plant compounds that includes flavonoids, in dried green tea leaf is 8% to 12%. Other compounds of interest in dried green tea leaf include the following:

- Caffeine (3.5%)
- Theanine (4%), an amino acid that can promote feelings of calmness while at the same time promoting mental clarity and focus

In order to gain the health benefits of green tea, a sufficient dosage of the polyphenols must be achieved. One study sought to determine the dose effect of green tea on antioxidant protection. In the study, fifteen healthy volunteers consumed 500 ml of green tea with different contents of solids (1.4, 1.6, 1.8, and 2.0 grams per liter). Ingestion of the lowest dosage produced no change in plasma antioxidant capacity. At the highest dosage, the effects increased the plasma antioxidant capacity the greatest at one and four hours after ingestion. This study is significant as it indicates that some of the studies failing to show health benefits of green tea ingestion may have been due to insufficient dosage.

In addition to exerting direct antioxidant activity on its own, green tea increases the activity of antioxidant enzymes within the body. The human antioxidant system involves not only the use of dietary compounds such as green tea polyphenols but also a number of enzymes produced by cells to deactivate damaging compounds. This effect is important because often nutritionists look only at the direct action of the food component as an antioxidant instead of at the total effect on the body's antioxidant system. The total antioxidant effects of green tea far exceed its direct antioxidant effects.

The same is true of green tea's anticancer effects. Yes, green tea polyphenols exert many direct anticancer actions, but they also have the ability to activate many of the body's own anticancer mechanisms. Population-based studies attest to the anticancer effects of green tea consumption. The forms of cancer that appear to be best prevented by green tea are those of the gastrointestinal tract, including the stomach, small intestine, pancreas, and colon; the lungs; estrogen-related cancers, including most breast cancers; skin cancer; and prostate cancer.

In addition to inhibition of the interaction of estrogen with its receptors in breast tissue, the polyphenol compounds in green tea block genetic factors that promote the interaction of tumor promoters, hormones, and growth factors with their receptors—a kind of sealing-off effect—in breast tissue. Experimental and epidemiologic studies have demonstrated a protective effect against breast cancer, and clinical results have confirmed that green tea might be helpful as a treatment for early stage breast cancer.

Interestingly, the best existing data on green tea's anticancer effects is on prostate cancer. Considerable evidence shows that the green tea polyphenol epigallocatechin gallate (EGCG) strongly inhibits all types of prostate cancer. Studies have shown that when men consume 6 cups of green tea daily or take an equivalent amount of green tea extract for four to six weeks before undergoing removal of their prostate (radical prostatectomy), EGCG is detectable in their blood and prostate tissue. Furthermore, in men taking green tea, numerous biomarkers of prostate cancer activity are dramatically impacted for the better. Even prostate-specific antigen (PSA) levels drop precipitously.

One of the strongest clinical studies showing the value of green tea in preventing prostate cancer involved evaluating the safety and efficacy of green tea polyphenols in men with a high-grade precancerous condition of the prostate.

The sixty men were given either a placebo or 600 mg of green tea polyphenol extract (GTPE) daily. After one year, only one tumor was diagnosed among the thirty GTPE-treated men, whereas nine cancers were found among the thirty placebo-treated men (incidence, 30%). Total PSA levels did not change significantly between the two groups of men, but GTPE-treated men showed values constantly lower with respect to those on the placebo. In addition, the International Prostate Symptom Score and quality-of-life scores of GTPE-treated men improved. Symptoms such as increased nighttime awakening to urinate, decreased caliber of urine flow, and feelings of urgency all improved with GTPE. These results suggest that GTPE might also be of help in treating the symptoms of benign prostate enlargement. All of these benefits were achieved without side effects.

Similar to studies on antioxidant activity, however, results seem to be dependent upon a sufficient dosage. In a study in men with precancerous prostate lesions, a dosage of 400 mg of EGCG per day for one year showed some benefit, but not to the same statistical significance as the higher dosage. In the EGCG group, five out of forty-nine subjects developed prostate cancer, compared to nine out of forty-eight taking the placebo. In addition, PSA levels were lowered only in the EGCG group. The takeaway is that in order to see a statistically significant effect in men with early stage prostate cancer, higher dosages of green tea or green tea extract have to be consumed, i.e., a minimum of 600 mg of total polyphenols per day. Getting that dosage of polyphenols from drinking green tea requires an intake of four to six cups daily.

Green Tea and Weight Loss

Green tea extracts have become a popular weight-loss aid. The desired effect appears to require both the polyphenols and caffeine. In one clinical trial, extracts containing both ingredients decreased body mass index (–0.55), body weight (–1.38 kg), and waist circumference (–1.93 cm). However, when either the polyphenols or caffeine was given alone in trials, they did not have much effect. Green tea catechin and caffeine mixtures promote weight loss through increasing the process of thermogenesis, which means that fat is burned in a way that increases heat production. To achieve a dosage similar to that used in the positive studies requires an intake of at least six cups of regular green tea (sencha, page 107) or an extract with a similar chemical profile that provides 300 mg of polyphenols and 150 mg of caffeine.

Theanine

A discussion of the health benefits of green tea would be incomplete if it did not highlight theanine, a major amino acid uniquely found in green tea. Theanine is used by the tea plant in the manufacture of its polyphenols during the process of photosynthesis. Theanine is also the compound responsible for the characteristic taste and aroma of green tea.

In regard to health benefits, theanine exerts many interesting effects, especially on brain chemistry. While it is true that caffeine is a stimulant and theanine buffers some of the effects of caffeine in the brain, it is wrong to think of theanine as a "downer." It is anything but that, as it stimulates brain energy, though in a different way from caffeine. In animal models, theanine has been shown to increase brain levels of many different brain chemicals, especially the neurotransmitters that carry signals from one brain cell to another. In these studies, it has definitely improved brain function, learning, and memory. Those findings may explain why theanine-rich green tea is so valued as an aid to meditation and revered in green tea ceremonies.

Theanine's effects on dopamine are particularly interesting, as this compound is central to the reward and pleasure sensations we experience. The immediate release of dopamine is one of the key reasons certain behaviors and drugs become addictive. Theanine seems to modify dopamine response and holds some promise in fighting certain kinds of addictions, such as those to nicotine and sugar.

Human clinical studies have confirmed many of the unique effects of theanine, which have been shown to reduce the negative side effects of caffeine, such as anxiety and irritability. It has also been shown to reduce stress, improve sleep quality, diminish premenstrual symptoms, heighten mental acuity, and provide some benefits in attention deficit/hyperactivity disorder.

One of the key effects of theanine's complex actions in the brain is an increase in the production of alpha brain waves. These are associated with feelings of calmness and focus. During meditation, an abundance of alpha brain waves is produced. Matcha, the form of green tea most valued by Japanese monks for their tea ceremony, is the richest source of theanine and contains only a modest amount of caffeine. Theanine accentuates the meditative state by promoting greater mental focus and alertness. In addition to boosting alpha brain waves, theanine decreases beta waves, which are associated with nervousness, scattered thoughts, and hyperactivity.

Theanine is a popular ingredient in functional foods and beverages as well as dietary supplements designed to produce mental and physical relaxation without inducing drowsiness. Theanine is fast acting; its effects are felt within the first thirty minutes and have been shown to last up to eight to twelve hours. Based on clinical studies, it has been established that theanine is effective in the range of 50 to 200 mg. Theanine is available as a dietary supplement.

As for green tea, gyokuro and matcha teas are known for having high amounts of theanine. These tea plants are put under shade during the last three weeks before harvest. The result is that less photosynthesis occurs so that more theanine is left in the leaves, giving gyokuro and matcha their characteristic sweetness and flavor. In the shade, chlorophyll is concentrated in the tips of the plants, resulting in leaves that are bright green in color. While standard green tea may have a theanine content as low as 5 mg per cup, shade-grown green tea may have as much as nine times this amount per cup, about 45 mg, but most often contains 25 to 30 mg per cup. As for caffeine content, gyokuro has the highest, at 160 mg per cup, while matcha comes in at a modest 30 mg per cup.

How Much Green Tea?

More than 150 varieties and grades of green tea are available as loose tea or in bags. Try different brands and types of green tea to find one that you enjoy. It is important to store your tea properly to prevent its deterioration. Place loose tea in a canister with a tight seal and store in a cupboard away from light. Consider transferring tea bags packaged in flimsy cardboard boxes and wrapped in paper to canisters or plastic bags. Properly stored green tea will keep up to a year. My favorite green teas are sencha and matcha.

- *Sencha*, the most popular of Japan's green teas, produces a clear yellowish green liquor with a sweet, grassy, lightly astringent flavor; the tea can vary dramatically in both price and quality. Lower-quality sencha tea is called *bancha*.

• *Matcha* is the tea used in the traditional Japanese tea ceremony. Matcha is unique in two areas: farming and processing. Like sencha, matcha is shade-grown for about three weeks before harvest. Prior to grinding the leaves into a fine powder, the stems and veins are removed, making matcha vibrant in both color and taste. Matcha comes in different grades based upon what part of the plant is used. Matcha produced from the tips of the leaves is regarded as the highest quality.

To brew green tea, rinse out an empty teapot and fill it with hot water. Boil freshly drawn tap water. If the quality of your tap water is poor, try using filtered or bottled spring water. In order to draw the best flavor out of the tea, heat the water to just below boiling. Empty the hot water from your teapot and add 1 rounded teaspoon tea leaves for each 6 ounces water. For maximum flavor, place the tea directly into the bottom of the pot or use a basket infuser. Tea ball strainers, though convenient, often yield poorer-tasting tea as they are often too small to allow all of the leaves to unravel fully. If you do use a tea ball, be sure to use one that is large so the tea can expand. Pour the freshly boiled water over the leaves in the teapot.

Steep the tea for 3 to 5 minutes. Tea becomes bitter if steeped for longer than 5 minutes. Remove the infuser and the tea. If you placed the tea directly into the pot, pour the tea into cups through a strainer to catch the leaves.

For iced green tea, pour 1 cup boiling water over two tea bags and let steep for 3 to 5 minutes. Remove and squeeze out the tea bags. Add ice and enjoy. Double or triple the amount to enjoy throughout the day.

For a hot tea punch with more flavonoid content, brew 5 bags of green tea in 6 cups water along with 2 cinnamon sticks and 8 whole cloves. Add 1½ cups orange juice and ⅓ cup fresh lemon juice. Serve hot.

To brew matcha tea properly, you will need some traditional utensils: a strainer and a bamboo whisk. Place a small strainer over a tea bowl and measure 3 teaspoons matcha powder into it. Gently tap the side of the strainer to sift the tea into the bowl. Pour 2 ounces of hot water just shy of boiling (165°

to 180°F/75° to 80°C) into a teacup. I recommend using purified water; ordinary tap water will result in tea that won't taste as good as it should. Pour half of the water into the tea bowl with the matcha powder and whisk rapidly with the bamboo whisk, using circular motions. Pour the rest of the water into the bowl and stir it with the bamboo whisk until the matcha paste thins out. Pour the tea into your cup and drink it immediately. If you wait too long, the matcha powder will settle to the bottom of the cup. Enjoy!

I recommend drinking 18 to 24 ounces of regular green tea daily or 6 to 8 ounces matcha.

4. Bee Pollen

Bees are essential to life, given their role in pollinating plants. Recently, there has been an alarming decline in bee numbers in North America due to a phenomenon known as colony collapse disorder (CCD). The suggested causes of CCD include pesticides, pathogens, and beekeeping practices, but no single factor has been consistently found to suggest that one thing in particular is the sole cause.

In addition to their role in pollination, bees provide us with some wondrous nutritional products, including honey and bee pollen. Bee pollen comes from the male germ cell of flowering plants. As the honeybee travels from flower to flower, it fertilizes the female germ cell. Honeybees enable the reproduction of more than 80% of the world's grains, fruits, vegetables, and legumes. The pollen is collected and brought to the hive, where the bees add enzymes and nectar. One teaspoon of bee pollen takes a single bee working eight hours a day one month to gather.

Little research has been done on bee pollen and other bee products, such as propolis and royal jelly, probably because the financial rewards to justify such an investment are lacking. The research that does exist is limited but impressive. Studies in animals show that pollen can promote growth and development; improve semen quality; increase fertility; protect against free-radical and oxidative damage; and protect against the effects of harmful radiation, as well as toxic exposure to chemical solvents. Clinical applications for bee products include allergies, antioxidant support, energy enhancement, menopausal symptoms, and support for chemotherapy and radiation therapy.

In a human study, a pollen extract showed significant improvement in menopausal symptoms (headache, urinary incontinence, dry vagina, decreasing vitality) in double-blind studies. The improvements were achieved even though the pollen extract produces no estrogenic effect, an important consideration for women who cannot take estrogens of any kind.

If you have a known allergy to pollen or conifer and poplar trees, the use of bee products should be avoided. Allergic reactions can range from mild gastrointestinal upset to severe reactions such as asthma, anaphylaxis (shock), intestinal bleeding, and even death in those who are allergic to bee products.

I find that taking 1 to 2 tablespoons bee pollen granules, rather than capsules or tablets, daily gives me higher energy levels. Bee pollen is a complete protein, meaning it contains all eight essential amino acids. In fact, bee pollen is higher in protein content than any animal source and about half of its protein is in the form of free amino acids that are ready to be used directly by the body. Bee pollen also provides significant levels of B vitamins, vitamin C, carotenes, minerals, DNA, RNA, numerous flavonoid molecules, and plant hormones.

Children under one year of age should not be given any honey or other bee products.

5. Ground Flaxseed

Flax (*Linum usitatissimum*) is a plant native to the Mediterranean but now grown in many places. The seeds can be ground to make a high-fiber meal or oil, also known as flaxseed or linseed oil. The plant's stems are used to make linen cloth. Flaxseeds, which are slightly larger than sesame seeds and have a hard shell that is smooth and shiny, range in color from deep amber to reddish brown depending whether the flax is of the golden or brown variety. Ground flaxseed can have a relatively slippery texture with a potential hint of crunch, depending upon how finely it is ground.

Flaxseed and flaxseed oil are the most abundant sources of lignans. These components are fiber compounds that can bind to estrogen receptors and interfere with the cancer-promoting effects of estrogen on breast tissue. Lignans also increase the production of a compound known as sex hormone binding globulin, or SHBG. This protein regulates estrogen levels by escorting excess estrogen from the body.

Population studies, as well as experimental studies in humans and animals, have demonstrated that lignans exert significant anticancer effects. In one study, researchers followed twenty-eight postmenopausal nuns for a year and tracked their blood levels of two cancer-related estrogens, estrone sulfate and estradiol. In addition to their normal diets, the nuns received daily supplements of 0, 5, or 10 grams of ground flaxseed. Estrogen levels fell significantly in the women taking ground flaxseed, but they remained stable in the control group (those taking no flaxseed). Reducing estrogen levels reduces breast cancer risk.

Dr. Paul Gross, director of the breast cancer prevention program at the Princess Margaret Hospital and the Toronto Hospital, has reported that flaxseed in the diet may shrink breast cancers. His study involved fifty women who had recently been diagnosed with breast cancer. While waiting for their surgery, the women were divided into two groups. One group received a daily muffin containing 25 grams (a little less than 2 tablespoons) of ground flaxseed. The others were prescribed ordinary muffins. After surgery, the investigators found that women who had received the flaxseed muffins had slower-growing tumors than the others.

Ground flaxseed has also been shown to be helpful in improving blood lipid profiles. In one double-blind trial, thirty-six postmenopausal women were given 40 grams (approximately 3 tablespoons) of either ground flaxseed or a wheat-based placebo daily for three months. In the women given ground flaxseed, total cholesterol blood levels dropped by 6%, but no reduction in cholesterol occurred in the women given wheat. In women on the flaxseed regimen, blood levels of both LDL ("bad") and HDL ("good") cholesterol dropped by 4.7%, and triglyceride levels dropped by 12.8%, resulting in only a minor reduction in the ratio of "bad" to "good" cholesterol. However, in the women given ground flaxseed, blood levels of two cholesterol-carrying molecules, apolipoprotein A-1 and apolipoprotein B, were reduced by 6% and 7.5%, respectively. Research suggests that these cholesterol-carrying molecules are better indicators of heart disease risk than cholesterol alone.

Flaxseed oil contains nearly twice the level of omega-3 fatty acids as fish oils—although it is the shorter-chain alpha-linolenic acid (ALA) rather than the longer-chain omega-3 fatty acids such as eicosapentaenoic acid (EPA) and docosahexaenoic acid (DHA). ALA can be converted to these but has itself shown benefits including reducing the risk of developing heart disease and cancer. Data derived from biopsies of breast fatty tissue at the time of diagnosis in women with breast cancer compared with women with benign breast disease indicated that the relative risk of breast cancer for women with higher breast tissue levels of ALA was 64% less than for those at the lowest level. In another study, the higher the level of ALA in breast tissue, the less likely the cancer was to spread into the lymph nodes of the armpit or be invasive.

Some studies indicate that ALA may increase the risk of prostate cancer. However, in some of these studies ALA intake was used as a marker for meat intake. In the absence of consuming vegetable sources of ALA such as flaxseed oil, the primary dietary source is from meat—the greater the meat intake, the higher the tissue ALA level. It is also possible that deficiencies of zinc or other nutrients involved in the conversion of ALA to EPA were ultimately responsible for the elevations in ALA levels noted in men with prostate cancer. About 50% of all men with prostate cancer are deficient in zinc.

No one has looked at the effect of flaxseed oil in prostate cancer. Ground flaxseed, however, appears to be helpful not only in preventing prostate cancer but also in treating men with existing prostate cancer. In addition to the phytoestrogen effect, flaxseed lignans bind to male hormone receptors and promote the elimination of testosterone. In a study conducted at the Duke University Medical Center and Durham Veterans Affairs Medical Center involving men with prostate cancer, a low-fat diet (in which fat represented no more than 20% of total calories) supplemented with 30 grams of ground flaxseed (roughly 2 tablespoons) reduced serum testosterone by 15%, slowed the growth rate of cancer cells, and increased the death rate of cancer cells after only thirty-four days.

Ground flaxseed is important when it comes to cardiovascular health due to its blood pressure–lowering effect. A study conducted at the St. Boniface Hospital Research Centre in Winnipeg, Canada, examined the effects of daily ingestion of ground flaxseed on systolic blood pressure (SBP) and diastolic blood pressure (DBP) in patients with peripheral artery disease. A total of 110 patients ingested a variety of foods that contained 30 grams of ground flax-seed or placebo each day over six months. Results included the plasma levels of alpha-linolenic acid and lignans increasing two- and fiftyfold, respectively, in the flaxseed-fed group but not in the placebo group. The subjects' body weights were not significantly different between the two groups at any time. The big changes occurred in blood pressure.

While individuals with normal BP showed no effect with six months of flaxseed ingestion, those patients who entered the trial with an SBP of ≥140 mm Hg at baseline obtained an average reduction of 15 mm Hg in SBP and 7 mm Hg in DBP. In other words, this major antihypertensive effect was achieved selectively in hypertensive patients. The benefits in lowering blood pressure are likely a combination of several nutritional factors in ground flax-seed. The bottom line is that this simple dietary intervention produced one of the most potent antihypertensive effects achieved by any dietary factor.

Ground flaxseed, also called flaxseed meal, is sold in health food and gro-cery stores. Once opened, store ground flaxseed in the refrigerator, because it can turn rancid at room temperature. The same is true of flaxseed oil; it must be refrigerated. Whole flaxseed must be ground to make it digestible and absorbable. Stir 2 tablespoons ground flaxseed daily into your oatmeal, smoothie, or yogurt.

6. Whey Protein

Whey is a natural by-product of the cheese-making process. Cow's milk has about 6.25% protein. Of that, 80% is casein (another type of protein) and the remaining 20% is whey. When cheese is made, it uses the casein molecules, leaving the whey behind. Whey protein is made via filtering off the other com-ponents of whey, such as lactose, fats, and minerals. It is soluble and easy to digest and is efficiently absorbed into the body. When taken prior to a meal, it improves blood sugar control.

Whey protein has the highest biological value of all proteins. In order to assess the quality of a protein, scientists measure the proportion of the amino acids that are absorbed, retained, and used in the body to determine the pro-tein's biological value (BV).

Whey protein is a complete protein in that it contains all essential and nonessential amino acids. One of the key reasons the BV of whey protein is so high is that it has the highest concentrations of glutamine and branched-chain amino acids (BCAAs) found in nature. Glutamine and branched-chain amino acids are essential to cellular health, muscle growth, and protein synthesis.

Glutamine, the most abundant amino acid in the body, is involved in more metabolic processes than any other amino acid. It is important as a source of fuel for white blood cells and for cells that divide rapidly, such as those that line the intestine. Supplementation with glutamine has been shown to heal peptic ulcers, enhance energy levels, boost immune function, and fight infections.

Although body builders and athletes use whey protein to increase their protein intake, almost everyone can gain benefit by adding it to his or her diet. Whey protein is especially important as an aid in weight loss, as nutritional support for recovery from surgery, and to offset some of the negative effects of radiation therapy and chemotherapy.

Research has shown that individuals who exercise benefit from diets high in the essential amino acid leucine and have more lean muscle tissue and less body fat than those whose diets contain lower levels of leucine. Whey protein concentrates have approximately 50% more leucine than does soy protein isolate.

Whey Protein, an Immune Function and Detoxification Aid

Whey protein has been shown to boost immune function by raising the levels of the important antioxidant glutathione, which is found in all cells, including white blood cells. Sufficient glutathione levels are essential to proper immune functioning. In immune cells, glutathione stimulates antibody production and the ability of white blood cells to engulf and destroy invading organisms.

Glutathione is also involved in the body's detoxification reactions and binds to fat-soluble toxins such as heavy metals, solvents, and pesticides, transforming them into a water-soluble form, allowing for more efficient excretion via the kidneys. Eating additional whey protein is one of the best ways to raise glutathione levels in the body and assist in effective detoxification.

Whey Protein Is a Dieter's Friend

Whey protein ingestion has been shown to reduce feelings of hunger and promote satiety, making it a valuable aid in weight-loss programs. It contains bioactive components that help stimulate the release of three appetite-suppressing gut hormones: cholecystokinin (CCK), peptide tyrosine-tyrosine (PYY), and glucagonlike peptide-1 (GLP-1).

One of the best strategies for utilizing whey protein is to take it before or between meals. Studies have shown that consumption of whey protein in small amounts prior to a meal improves after-meal blood sugar control and also leads to greater satiety and appetite control. By stabilizing blood sugar levels and reducing hunger, dieting is easier and success more likely.

Vegan sources of whey protein do not seem to be able to duplicate these weight-loss benefits. In a study conducted at the University of Birmingham in the United Kingdom, forty overweight men and women completed a fourteen-day calorie restricted diet and were randomly assigned, double blind, to receive twice-daily supplements of isolated whey (27 grams), soy (26 grams), or maltodextrin (25 grams). A blood measurement of muscle fiber synthesis indicated that muscle breakdown was significantly less in the whey protein group than that seen in the soy and maltodextrin groups. In fact, soy protein had no effect on reducing muscle loss. These results indicate that whey protein supplementation can help preserve muscle mass during weight loss.

Fight Aging by Increasing Muscle Mass with Diet, Whey Protein, and Exercise

One of the most preventable changes associated with aging is the loss of muscle mass and strength, which is called sarcopenia. Sarcopenia is to muscle mass what osteoporosis is to bones. While osteoporosis gets all the media attention, sarcopenia is a more significant factor. The degree of sarcopenia is the major predictor of physical disability and is linked to decreased vitality, poor balance, walking speed, falls, and fractures, especially among elderly people.

Just as building strong bones when young is important in preventing osteoporosis later in life, building and maintaining muscle mass is essential for avoiding sarcopenia. Muscle mass increases throughout childhood and peaks during the late teens through the mid to late 20s. After that, a slow decline in muscle mass begins. From the age of 25 to 50 the decline in muscle mass is roughly 10%. In our fifties the rate of decline is slightly accelerated, but the real decline usually begins at age 60. By the time a person reaches 80, his or her muscle mass is a little more than half of what it was in the twenties. Taking whey protein, engaging in weight-bearing exercises, and lifting weights can help preserve muscle mass and can even help those with sarcopenia rebuild.

The amount of whey protein you need depends on how active you are. If you are active and work out regularly, I recommend taking 50 grams of whey protein daily. If you exercise infrequently, then take 25 grams per day.

You can find whey protein powder in a variety of flavors, including vanilla, chocolate, and strawberry, available in premeasured individual serving packets and bulk containers. Usually these protein powders are found in the body-building sections of health food stores. The highest quality is often referred to as microfiltered or ultrafiltered.

7. Soluble Dietary Fiber Supplements

The health benefits of water-soluble dietary fiber—found in most fruits and vegetables, legumes, oat bran, pectin, and psyllium husks—are immense. In addition to a diet rich in fruits and vegetables, I highly recommend including a source of additional dietary fiber into your diet. The best choices are PGX®, psyllium seed husks (e.g., Metamucil), guar gum, pectin, and resistant dextrin (e.g., tapioca fiber). Personally, I take PolyGlycopleX (PGX), a viscous, soluble fiber as a dietary supplement. PGX is produced by a patented process that allows three natural fibers (konjac root, alginate, and xanthan gum) to coalesce and form a matrix that has a higher level of viscosity, gel-forming properties, and more expansion when combined with water than any other soluble fiber source. In essence, PGX is a "super fiber" with all of the beneficial effects of dietary fiber, but magnified and more easily achieved. It is especially helpful in promoting the feeling of satiety (fullness) when taken before meals.

Clinical studies with soluble dietary fiber supplements have shown them to produce the following benefits:

- Increase the level of compounds that block the appetite and promote satiety

- Decrease the level of compounds that stimulate overeating

- Reduce the glycemic index of any food, beverage, or meal (by as much as 70%)

- Increase insulin sensitivity and promote improved blood sugar control

- Help stabilize blood sugar levels to reduce food cravings

In my opinion, soluble dietary fiber supplements are one of the most important natural products available today because of their ability to address the core underlying reasons why weight loss and blood sugar control are often so difficult to achieve. These supplements are available in granules, capsules, drink mixes, and weight-loss meal replacement formulas. Regardless of the form, the usual dosage recommendation for soluble dietary fiber is 2.5 to 5 grams before meals.

Since dietary fiber supplements can slow down or interfere with the absorption of drugs, be sure to take any medications at least one hour before or after taking any dietary fiber supplement and consult with your doctor.

While I am passionate about these seven superfoods and make them a big part of my daily meals and snacks, remember to eat and drink a wide range of healthy foods for better health, higher energy levels, and greater clarity of thought.

7

Spice It Up!

Using more herbs, spices, and other seasonings to add flavor to food significantly improves our diet and health and fights disease.

What is the difference between a spice and an herb? Technically, an herb is a plant that does not have a woody stem. If a plant has a woody stem, it is referred to as a shrub, bush, or tree. The term *herb* is also used to describe a plant or plant part that is used for medicinal purposes. A spice, on the other hand, technically describes a plant product that has aromatic properties and is used to season or flavor foods.

Herbs used in cooking are composed of leaves and stems. This makes for an easy way of distinguishing herbs from spices, as most spices are derived from bark, for example cinnamon; fruit, for example red and black pepper; seed, for example nutmeg; or other parts of herbs, trees, and shrubs.

Garlic, ginger, salt, and other flavor enhancers are classified as seasonings since they don't have the characteristics of herbs and spices.

When using herbs, fresh ones are always preferred over dried for their health benefits and the distinct flavors they add to foods. To prepare most fresh herbs for use, first remove the stems, then put the leaves into a measuring cup. With your kitchen shears, mince them to the desired size.

If using a recipe that calls for dried herbs but you only have fresh, use four times as much of the fresh one. For example, to season enough vegetables for four servings, start with 1 teaspoon minced fresh herbs or ¼ teaspoon crushed dried herbs. Taste and then add more as needed. Dried herbs and spices should be stored in a cool dark place away from heat and sunlight. Most ground spices should be used within six months; whole ones will keep for a year. Before using them, smell dried herbs and spices for freshness. If they have no aroma or smell like dried grass, replace them. In this book, spices come first, followed by herbs and then seasonings. Whichever ones you choose to cook with, know that they pack a powerful punch of antioxidant activity. They also activate the enzyme AMPk, which is so important in promoting weight loss and fighting the aging process. Use them frequently and liberally.

The Magic of Spices

Black Pepper

Pepper is the most widely used spice in the world and deservedly so. The tropical pepper plant produces a black fruit (peppercorn). There are two basic types available.

- With its black skin left intact, black pepper is the most pungent and flavorful of all types of peppers. Black pepper is available whole, cracked, or ground into a powder.

- White pepper is produced by removing the outer black skin of the peppercorn and tastes more aromatic, with less bite than black pepper. White pepper is available whole, cracked, or ground into a powder.

Health Benefits

Black pepper has been valued primarily in the treatment of digestive disorders. It stimulates the taste buds and causes an increase in stomach acid secretion, thereby improving digestion. In addition, it is a carminative, a substance that helps prevent the formation of intestinal gas.

Black pepper has diaphoretic (promotes sweating) and diuretic (promotes urination) properties. Not only does it help you derive the most benefit from

your food, it stimulates the breakdown of fat cells. Many of its health benefits
are due to the pungent compound piperine, which has been shown to:

- Dramatically increase the absorption of certain nutrients, such as selenium, B vitamins, and beta-carotene, as well as various herbal compounds and drugs

- Support and assist the body's fat-burning mechanisms

- Support and enhance the liver's detoxification processes

- Possibly be helpful in neurological disorders, including epilepsy, Par
  kinson's disease, depression, and pain

- Possibly help reverse important mechanisms that lead to resistance to
  antibiotics and anticancer drugs

Experimental studies designed to assess the toxicity of black pepper
showed that when rats or mice were given black pepper as a major part of
their diet, they thrived and their life span increased dramatically compared to
the control group. For example, when 5% of their diet was made up of black
pepper, they lived 20% longer than mice on the control diet. In another study,
mice injected with a type of tumor and then fed black pepper had a life span
that was 64% longer than that of mice not given the black pepper.

When researchers asked why black pepper is so effective in increasing
life span, the answers pointed to black pepper's antioxidant- and detoxifica-
tion-enhancing effects. For example, piperine and other black pepper components have been shown to activate the liver enzyme glutathione-S-transferase.
This enzyme helps attach the antioxidant molecule glutathione to toxic molecules that would otherwise do damage in the body. This action makes black
pepper a "chemoprotective" food that can help neutralize particular types
of carcinogens, such as the benzopyrenes that are found in cigarette smoke,
charcoal-grilled foods, and most other sources of smoke. The bottom line is
that if you can protect cells in the body, especially the liver, from chemical

assault and at the same time enhance their ability to eliminate harmful substances, they will function better and live longer. Liberally grind black peppercorns onto your food.

Using Black Pepper

Since the aromatic oils in peppercorns lose their flavor and aroma if heated for too long, grind whole peppercorns in a pepper mill just before adding to food. In addition to their superior flavor, buying whole peppercorns will help ensure that you are purchasing unadulterated pepper, since ground pepper is often mixed with other spices.

Whole peppercorns will keep in a cool, dark, dry place almost indefinitely, while ground pepper loses its potency after a few weeks.

- Wrap about 10 whole peppercorns in cheesecloth and immerse the package into soups and stews while cooking. Be sure to remove the package before serving.

- The pairing of black pepper and vanilla is surprisingly delicious. To experience and enjoy this flavor combination, mix freshly ground black pepper into vanilla-flavored foods such as yogurt, ice milk, cakes, or sauces.

Cayenne Pepper

Cayenne, or red pepper (*Capsicum frutescens*), is the fruit of *Capsicum annuum longum*, a shrubby tropical plant that can grow to a height of up to 3 feet. The fruit is technically a berry; it is usually 1 to 2 cm in diameter and can vary from 1 to 12 cm in length. Cayenne and most other *Capsicum* varieties range from moderately to very spicy. Paprika, however, is a milder, sweeter-tasting fruit produced from a different variety of *Capsicum annuum*.

Cayenne peppers, as well as other chile peppers, can trace their seven-thousand-year history to Central and South America. In those areas, cayenne peppers were used first as a decorative item and then as a food and medicine.

Capsaicin, although hot to the taste, has been shown to lower body temperature by stimulating the cooling center of the hypothalamus in the brain. The ingestion of cayenne peppers by people native to the tropics appears to offer a way for people living in those areas to get relief from high temperatures. How "cool" is that?

Health Benefits

The intense heat of cayenne peppers is produced by their high concentration of capsaicin. This compound is well recognized in clinical research as an effective pain reliever, as a digestive and antiulcer aid, and for its cardiovascular benefits. The fruit of this plant has the ability to cool body temperatures, especially in regions of intense tropical heat. Capsaicin is also the component responsible for cayenne pepper's ability to increase basal metabolic rate and stimulate the burning of fat for energy.

Capsaicin is responsible for the irritating effect of red pepper when it is applied to the skin or ingested via its ability to cause the release of substance P (the "P" stands for pain) from nerve cells, which in turn results in irritation and pain. Once substance P is released, capsaicin works to block its reuptake. The result is that repeated applications of capsaicin deplete substance P from small nerve fibers, thereby eventually blocking the pain sensation. A similar thing happens with the ingestion of cayenne pepper: the more frequently it is consumed, the greater the tolerance developed. In other words, the more red pepper you eat, the less spicy it becomes.

Capsaicin-containing creams and gels are available as FDA-approved topical treatments for arthritis and pain caused by diabetic neuropathy. Clinical studies demonstrate that capsaicin products applied topically have shown impressive results in cases of psoriasis, rheumatoid arthritis, and postherpes pain (postherpetic neuralgia). Topical capsaicin preparations have also been shown to be an effective treatment for cluster headaches and osteoarthritic pain.

Cayenne pepper exerts beneficial effects internally, such as stimulating and enhancing digestion. A study published in *The New England Journal of Medicine* found that daily doses of red pepper significantly reduced symptoms of indigestion in individuals with frequent indigestion (functional dyspepsia). In this placebo-controlled trial, thirty men and women with frequent indigestion were randomly assigned to receive either 2.5 grams of red pepper powder three times a day before meals or a placebo for five weeks. (Individuals who had been diagnosed with gastroesophageal reflux disease [GERD] or irritable bowel syndrome were excluded from the study.) Each day during the trial, the study participants scored and recorded the severity of their symptoms, such as stomach pain, stomach fullness, nausea, and changes in appetite. At the end of the trial, those who had been given red pepper powder were found to have fewer or less severe symptoms than those who received the placebo. In the group receiving red pepper, nausea, stomach pain, stomach fullness, and overall symptom scores were 38%, 50%, 46%, and 48% lower, respectively, than those of the placebo group.

Some evidence supports the idea that spicy foods containing cayenne and turmeric may help heal peptic ulcers. Specifically, double-blind studies have shown that red pepper consumption protects against aspirin-induced stomach damage and improves abdominal pain, fullness, and nausea scores in people with nonulcer dyspepsia. Nonetheless, some people are definitely bothered by ingestion of cayenne pepper as it may lower their threshold for heartburn.

Cayenne pepper also has beneficial effects on the cardiovascular system. Specifically, it reduces the likelihood of developing atherosclerosis, by reducing blood cholesterol and triglyceride levels and platelet aggregation, as well as by increasing fibrinolytic activity. Fibrinolytic activity is the ability to prevent the formation of blood clots, which can lead to a heart attack, stroke, or pulmonary embolism. Populations that consume large amounts of cayenne pepper have much lower rates of these diseases and conditions.

Finally, several studies have shown that increasing the intake of cayenne pepper may be an effective method to increase the basal metabolic rate and the burning of fat for energy (lipid oxidation). In the most recent study, after ingesting a standardized dinner on the previous evening, the subjects ate one of the following for breakfast: a high-fat meal including red pepper (10 grams), a high-carbohydrate meal, or a high-carbohydrate meal including red pepper (10 grams). The burning of fat for energy was significantly enhanced by the addition of red pepper to either meal, but especially the high-fat meal. Adding hot peppers to your diet is a safe, natural way to enhance fat burning.

Using Cayenne Peppers

Cayenne peppers are available as whole fresh or dried, crushed dried, or ground. Paprika is available dried and ground. If you grind your own peppers, take care not to inhale any dust, which can be irritating to the nasal passages and lungs.

Ground cayenne peppers and paprika can be kept in a sealed glass jar, away from direct sunlight, for up to one year.

- Keep a container of cayenne pepper on the table to spice up food.

- Add a pinch of cayenne pepper to hot cocoa for a Mexican flair.

- A dash of cayenne pepper will spice up bean dishes.

- Add cayenne to taste to 2 tablespoons lemon juice and stir into 3 cups cooked collard greens, mustard greens, or kale.

- To make your own chili powder (not ground chiles), stir together 2 tablespoons paprika, ½ teaspoon ground cayenne, 1 tablespoon ground turmeric, ½ teaspoon dried oregano, ⅛ teaspoon ground cumin, ⅛ teaspoon ground coriander, ⅛ teaspoon garlic powder, and ¼ teaspoon ground ginger.

Cinnamon

Cinnamon comes from the inner bark of evergreen trees native to southwest India and Asia. Once peeled away from the tree, the brown bark curls up into tubular "sticks," called quills, as it dries. Cinnamon and its oil are used as a flavoring agent in pharmaceutical, personal health, and cosmetic products. Cinnamon is available either as cinnamon sticks or as ground powder.

Health Benefits

Cinnamon has a long history in both Eastern and Western cultures as a medicine for arthritis, asthma, cancer, diarrhea, fever, heart problems, insomnia, menstrual problems, peptic ulcers, psoriasis, and spastic muscles. There are scientific studies to support some of these uses, but the most popular use of cinnamon in modern medicine is in supporting blood sugar control. The beneficial compounds in this application are believed to be its water-soluble polyphenol components.

Up to 2015, eight clinical trials with cinnamon powder in patients with type 2 diabetes and an additional two studies in patients with prediabetes had been done. The dosage ranged from 500 mg to 6 grams per day for a duration of forty days to four months. Although not all of the research on cinnamon in patients with type 2 diabetes has shown an effect, the majority of studies with well-defined use, especially at higher dosage levels (equivalent to 1 teaspoon or 6 grams of crude cinnamon powder per day) have shown some benefits. For example, in one of the first studies, in sixty people with type 2 diabetes, 1 to 6 grams of cinnamon taken daily for forty days reduced fasting blood glucose levels by 18% to 29%, triglyceride levels by 23% to 30%, LDL ("bad") cholesterol levels by 7% to 27%, and total cholesterol levels by 12% to 26%.

The bottom line is that cinnamon and cinnamon extracts can help; their use should therefore be encouraged in those with type 2 diabetes. Cinnamon, however, is not likely to be a magic bullet on its own, and additional support with diet, lifestyle, and proper supplementation is necessary.

Using Cinnamon

- Add ground cinnamon to chicken dishes, curries, and fruit, particularly apples and pears.
- When poaching chicken or fish, add 2 cinnamon sticks to the liquid.
- Add ½ teaspoon ground cinnamon to black beans to use in burritos or nachos.

Cloves

Cloves (*Eugenia caryophyllus*) are the unopened flower buds of the clove tree. They must be hand harvested. Their flavor can be overpowering, so use small amounts of whole or ground cloves.

Health Benefits

Cloves contain significant amounts of an active component called eugenol, which has made them the subject of numerous health studies. Some studies show benefit for the prevention of toxicity from environmental pollutants, such as carbon tetrachloride; prevention of digestive tract cancers; and treatment of joint inflammation.

In the United States, eugenol extracts from cloves are used in dentistry in conjunction with root canal procedures, temporary fillings, and general gum pain. Eugenol and other components of cloves, including beta-caryophyllene, combine to work as a mild anesthetic and an antibacterial agent. For these beneficial effects, clove oil can be found in over-the-counter sore throat sprays and mouthwashes.

Using Cloves

- Sprinkle ⅛ teaspoon ground cloves and 1 teaspoon ground cinnamon in a cup of hot apple cider.
- Add a pinch of clove powder to your ground coffee before brewing.
- Pierce an onion with 5 or 6 whole cloves and add to soups, broths, or poaching liquids while cooking.
- Add clove powder, walnuts, and raisins to Thanksgiving stuffing.

Cumin

Cumin seed (*Cuminum cyminum*) possesses a powerful flavor described as penetrating and peppery with slight citrus overtones. Cumin's unique complexity provides a hallmark flavor to Mexican, Indian, and Middle Eastern dishes.

Health Benefits

Like other sources of aromatic compounds, cumin seeds have long been noted to be beneficial to the digestive system. Research in animals has indicated that cumin may stimulate the secretion of pancreatic enzymes, important factors in proper digestion and nutrient assimilation.

Cumin seeds may also have anticancer properties. In one study, cumin was shown to protect laboratory animals from developing stomach or liver tumors. This cancer-protective effect may be due to its potent free radical–scavenging abilities, as well as its ability to enhance the liver's detoxification enzymes.

Using Cumin

- For the best flavor, toast whole cumin seeds in a skillet over low heat for a minute or two, just until fragrant.

- Put 2 teaspoons cumin seeds in a mug, cover with 2 cups hot water, and steep for 5 minutes for a soothing tea.

- Stir 2 teaspoons cumin seeds, ½ cup diced dried apricots, 1 cup almonds, 2 tablespoons extra-virgin olive oil, and ½ teaspoon salt substitute into 2 cups of cooked brown rice.

- To make black bean soup, sauté 1 cup chopped onions, 1 cup sliced carrots, and ½ cup seeded chopped red bell pepper in 1 tablespoon extra-virgin olive oil. Stir in ¼ cup lime juice and 1 tablespoon ground cumin. Add 1 (15-ounce) can black beans, rinsed and drained, and 2 cups water. Bring to a boil and simmer for 3 minutes. Garnish each serving with a wedge of lime and a sprinkling of finely chopped fresh cilantro.

Mustard

Mustard seeds are an underutilized spice and condiment. Mustard plants are cruciferous vegetables related to broccoli, brussels sprouts, and cabbage. There are three principal types of mustard seeds: black mustard (*Brassica nigra*), white mustard (*Brassica alba*), and brown mustard (*Brassica juncea*). Black mustard seeds have the strongest flavor, while white mustard seeds (which have a yellowish color) are the mildest and are used to make American yellow mustard. Brown mustard seeds have a darker yellow color.

Dijon and yellow mustard have different flavor profiles, but they are both made with water and vinegar. Turmeric is added to yellow mustard to brighten the color. Mustard seeds are frequently used in Indian cooking.

Health Benefits

Like other cabbage-family vegetables, mustard contains plentiful amounts of phytochemicals called glucosinolates and isothiocyanates. These compounds have been extensively studied for their anticancer effects.

Using Mustard

- To make honey-mustard dressing, combine ⅓ cup extra-virgin olive oil, ⅓ cup white vinegar, ¼ cup prepared yellow mustard, and 1 tablespoon honey in a jar. Add a pinch of salt substitute, if desired. Put on the lid and shake well before using.

- Coat salmon fillets with Dijon mustard, cover, and marinate overnight in the refrigerator before cooking.

- This may sound crazy, but I dip vegetables such as sliced daikon radish into Dijon mustard. It is phenomenal for stuffed sinuses!

Nutmeg

Nutmeg (*Myristica fragrans*) is the seed of a tropical evergreen tree native to the Moluccas, the central Spice Islands of Indonesia. Like apricots, plums, and peaches, the nutmeg contains a hard, oval-shaped shiny brown stone, about 1¼ inches in length and ¾ inch in diameter. It is this seed that is dried and sold whole or ground as nutmeg.

Health Benefits

Nutmeg has long been used as a carminative to prevent intestinal gas formation and flatulence. Modern research has shown that nutmeg can be an effective antidiarrheal agent, reducing the amount of stool, increasing the period between evacuations, and improving intestinal tone while inhibiting the contractions that would normally be stimulated by irritating agents. In addition, nutmeg's demonstrated sedative effects have no harmful effects on blood pressure.

Nutmeg contains myristicin, an essential oil. When ingested in large amounts, it acts as a potent hallucinogenic with unpleasant side effects, including severe headache, cramps, extreme nausea, and, for frequent users, liver toxicity. No need to worry, though—the small amount of nutmeg dusted over a cup of eggnog or added to a savory stew, elegant vegetable dish, or festive dessert is too small to do anything but enhance your food.

In the nutmeg trade, broken nutmegs that have been infested by pests are referred to as "BWP" (broken, wormy, and punky) grade. Although BWP-grade nutmegs are legally allowed to be used only for distillation of oil of nutmeg and extraction of nutmeg oleoresin, they are ground and sold illegally. Since molds can produce aflatoxin (a highly carcinogenic compound) on BWP nuts, purchase whole nutmegs and grind them as needed.

Using Nutmeg

- Add freshly grated nutmeg at the end of the cooking process, since heat, which promotes the evaporation of its essential oils, diminishes its flavor.

- Nutmeg is used in mulling spices, baked or stewed fruit, curries, custards, and cooked vegetables. Grind a bit over spinach, potatoes, squash, sweet potatoes, carrots, broccoli, or cauliflower.

- For a pumpkin casserole, combine 2 cups 100% pumpkin puree; 2 cored, seeded, finely chopped apples; 2 cups chopped pineapple; ½ cup broken walnuts; 1 teaspoon ground cinnamon; ¼ teaspoon ground cloves; and ½ teaspoon nutmeg. Spoon it into a baking dish, cover, and bake at 350°F for 40 minutes.

Saffron

Saffron is the delicate red stigma (the female part of the flower, which catches pollen) of a small purple crocus (*Crocus sativus*) with grasslike leaves and purple flowers. The saffron crocus, a member of the lily family, generally flowers in the fall. In a good year, each plant can produce several flowers, each of which contains three bright red stigmas joined to a pale yellow stylus. To produce saffron, the stigmas must be painstakingly harvested by hand. The stigmas are then laid on mesh nets and dried to deepen their flavor. This labor-intensive process is what makes saffron the most expensive spice in the world. Once cured, saffron stigmas look like pieces of fine red-orange thread. More than five thousand flowers must be harvested to yield a single ounce of the spice.

Health Benefits

Historically, saffron has been used as an aphrodisiac, diaphoretic (to cause sweating), carminative (to prevent gas), and emmenagogue (to bring on menstruation). In Japan, saffron is encapsulated and used as a sleep aid and in the treatment of Parkinson's disease. Modern research suggests that the spice may provide protection against cancer, memory loss, heart disease, and inflammation. The most compelling research with saffron is as an antidepressant.

Using Saffron

- Add a pinch of ground saffron to any tomato-based fish soup or stew.
- Saffron is essential in two Spanish dishes: paella, a baked dish of long-grain rice and seafood or chicken, and arroz con pollo (chicken with rice).

Turmeric

Turmeric (*Curcuma longa*) is a member of the ginger family that is extensively cultivated in India, China, Indonesia, and other tropical countries. Like ginger, the rhizome (root) is the part that is utilized. In the past, turmeric powder was referred to as "Indian saffron" as its deep yellow-orange color is reminiscent of that of saffron. Turmeric is the major ingredient of curry powder and is also used in prepared mustard as a coloring agent. It is extensively used in a variety of foods for both its color and its flavor.

Health Benefits

Turmeric has long been a key component of both the Chinese and Indian systems of medicine. Modern research has focused on curcumin, turmeric's yellow pigment. Curcumin has been the subject of more than eight thousand published scientific studies over the last twenty years. Most of these studies have focused on its anti-inflammatory and anticancer effects in experimental models. Turmeric's anti-inflammatory effects on arthritis and pain have been shown to be comparable to those of drugs such as ibuprofen without significant toxic effects (ulcer formation, decreased white blood cell count, intestinal bleeding).

Some of its anti-inflammatory action is related to its antioxidant activity. Curcumin is particularly helpful in preventing LDL cholesterol from becoming oxidized and damaging arteries. It exerts other effects that are beneficial in preventing atherosclerosis (hardening of the arteries), including lowering of cholesterol levels, prevention of plaque formation, and prevention of the formation of blood clots by inhibiting platelet aggregation.

The anticancer effects of turmeric and curcumin have been demonstrated at all steps of cancer formation: initiation, promotion, and progression. Curcumin acts to protect against damage to DNA. This effect was recently demonstrated in a study in a community with a high content of groundwater arsenic. This metal, arsenic, is highly carcinogenic because it causes severe oxidative damage to DNA. Subjects' blood samples prior to curcumin supplementation showed severe DNA damage with increased levels of free radicals and lipid peroxidation. Three months of curcumin intervention reduced the DNA damage, retarded free-radical formation and lipid peroxidation, and raised the level of antioxidant activity. Some of curcumin's other preventive effects against cancer formation include the ability to:

- Inhibit the formation of cancer-causing nitrosamines
- Enhance the body's production of cancer-fighting compounds, such as glutathione
- Promote the liver's detoxification of cancer-causing compounds
- Prevent overproduction of cyclooxygenase 2 (COX-2), an enzyme that may contribute to the development of tumors

There is considerable evidence that curcumin protects against age-related brain damage and in particular Alzheimer's disease. Researchers began exploring this effect after noting that elderly (aged 70 to 79) residents of rural India who eat large amounts of turmeric have been shown to have the lowest incidence of Alzheimer's disease in the world: 4.4 times lower than that of Americans.

Using Turmeric

Turmeric is available as a whole fresh rhizome, like ginger, or as a ground powder. Fresh turmeric should be crisp and free of dark spots; it can be kept in the refrigerator for one month. Peel the fresh turmeric and use a Microplane rasp to grate it. Dried turmeric should be stored like other spices—in a cool, dark place—and used within a few months.

Since turmeric's deep yellow-orange color can easily stain, avoid getting it on clothing. To avoid a stain on the skin, quickly wash any affected area with soap and plenty of water. It might be a good idea to wear latex gloves when preparing foods with turmeric.

- Fresh turmeric can be juiced with other fruits and vegetables.

- To make curry powder, stir together 1 tablespoon ground cumin, 1 tablespoon ground ginger, 1 teaspoon fenugreek, 1 teaspoon fennel seed, 1 teaspoon ground ginger, 1 teaspoon ground turmeric, and 1½ teaspoons ground coriander.

- Stir ½ to 1 teaspoon ground turmeric into cooked legumes, particularly lentils or rice.

- Give salad dressings an orange-yellow hue by adding some ground turmeric to them.

The Magic of Herbs

As mentioned, use fresh herbs whenever possible. Many herbs in the mint family—mint, basil, rosemary—are available fresh in grocery stores and at farmers' markets. Wrap them in paper towels and store in the refrigerator. Use them quickly and frequently.

Mint

The mint family is one of the most useful medicinal and culinary herb families. The hairlike oil glands on the surfaces of the leaves and stems of the plants release the herb's essential oil. The herbs you probably use most commonly—basil, marjoram, oregano, peppermint, rosemary, sage, savory, thyme—are all members of the mint family.

Health Benefits

Like other aromatic plants, mint has long been used as carminatives, as digestants, and to relieve the gastrointestinal tract of spasms and gas. Taking an enteric-coated peppermint oil capsule has been shown to be effective in relieving symptoms of irritable bowel syndrome. (Enteric coating prevents the herb's oil from being released in the stomach before reaching the bowel.) Peppermint oil relaxes smooth muscle. Once the smooth muscles surrounding the intestine are relaxed, there is less chance of spasm and the indigestion that can accompany it. The menthol contained in peppermint may be a key reason for this bowel-comforting effect.

The volatile oils in mint, such as menthol, thymol, and carvacrol, exert antimicrobial effects. A clinical study in Mexico found oregano to be more effective against the infection-causing amoeba *Giardia lamblia* than the commonly used prescription drug tinidazole. Thymol and carvacrol have also been shown to inhibit the growth of bacteria, including *Pseudomonas aeruginosa* and *Staphylococcus aureus*, two bacteria that are often the cause of impetigo (an infection of the skin).

Historically, rosemary, also a member of the mint family, was believed to stimulate and strengthen the memory. One interesting line of research indicates that the volatile oils in mint may help improve brain function. In studies on aging in rats, thymol was found to significantly increase the percentage of healthy fats found in cell membranes and other cell structures. In particular, the amount of DHA (docosahexaenoic acid, an omega-3 fatty acid) in brain, kidney, and heart cell membranes increased. In other studies looking more closely at changes in brain cells, researchers found that the maximum benefits of thyme occurred when the food was introduced early in the rats' life cycle but was less effective in offsetting the problems of brain cell aging when introduced later. The possible human application of this research is to use thyme as a method to raise DHA levels in children with attention deficit disorder and possibly improve this condition. This effect would apply to all mint-family members.

Using True Mint

- Fresh or dried peppermint, spearmint, apple mint, or any other mint variety can be used to make tea. Put ¼ cup leaves and stems into a cup, cover with hot water, and steep for a few minutes; remove the mint before drinking.

- Green salads, marinated vegetables, corn, broccoli, asparagus, and legumes can be enhanced with a few tablespoons chopped fresh mint.

- In a pitcher, combine 1 cup chopped fresh mint leaves, the juice of 2 limes, and ¼ cup cane sugar. Stir in 2 quarts sparkling water to make a nonalcoholic mojito.

- Toss 2 cups cooked eggplant cubes with ½ cup chopped fresh mint leaves, ½ cup plain yogurt, 1 minced garlic clove, and ⅛ teaspoon cayenne.

- Combine ½ fennel bulb, sliced; ¼ sliced red onion; the sections of 1 peeled orange; and ¼ cup chopped fresh mint leaves in a salad.

- Sprinkle chopped mint leaves on fruit salad.

Using Basil

- Puree 1 cup chopped fresh basil, 2 to 3 garlic cloves, 1 to 2 tablespoons walnuts, and 2 to 3 tablespoons extra-virgin olive oil in a blender or food processor. Use this dairy-free pesto on pasta, grilled salmon, or whole wheat bruschetta or in soups.

- Add chopped fresh basil, particularly Thai basil, to stir-fries, especially those that include eggplant, cabbage, chile peppers, tofu, coconut milk, and cashew nuts.

- Steep ¼ cup chopped fresh basil leaves in 2 cups hot water for 8 minutes, covered, for tea.

Using Oregano and Marjoram

- Sprinkle mushrooms and onions sautéed in 1 tablespoon olive oil with some chopped marjoram and oregano leaves.

- Fold in the chopped herbs when whisking eggs to make frittatas or omelets.

Using Rosemary

- Remove the leaves from the rosemary stems and add to chicken and lamb dishes.

- Put a spring or two into the pot when making tomato sauces and soups.

- Puree ¼ cup fresh rosemary leaves with 3 tablespoons extra-virgin olive oil and use as a dipping sauce for bread.

Using Sage

- To make stuffing, combine 3 cups cubed whole grain bread, ½ cup extra-virgin olive oil, ¼ cup vegetable or chicken broth, ¼ cup water, 1 tablespoon chopped fresh sage leaves, 1½ teaspoons chopped fresh thyme, and ¼ teaspoon salt substitute. Pour into a baking dish, cover, and bake at 350°F for 30 minutes.

- For a refreshing salad, combine 2 cups seeded, sliced bell peppers, ½ medium sliced cucumber, ½ sliced sweet onion, 1 cup plain yogurt, and 2 tablespoons chopped fresh sage leaves.

Using Thyme

- Add 2 to 3 thyme sprigs to the pot when cooking beans or soups.

- Make a savory topping for grilled or baked fish by adding thyme and rosemary pesto: chop enough fresh thyme and rosemary to cover half the surface of the fish. Add equal parts chopped walnuts to the herbs. Season with salt and pepper. Smear on top of the fish and grill or bake.

Cilantro and Coriander

Coriander (*Coriandrum sativum*) is a bright green annual herb with slender, erect, and hollow stems. It is considered both an herb and a spice since both its leaves and its seeds are used as seasoning condiments. The parts of the plant used include the leaves and the dried ripe fruits, which are known as coriander seeds. Fresh coriander leaves are known as cilantro, and they bear a strong likeness to Italian flat-leaf parsley; both of them belong to the Umbelliferae family.

Health Benefits

The essential oils in the seeds make them an effective carminative and digestive aid. Modern scientific investigations of coriander have focused on its antimicrobial properties, antianxiety action, and cholesterol-lowering effects. These preliminary studies in animals confirm many of its historical uses. Its cholesterol-lowering action is the result of coriander stimulating the conversion of cholesterol to bile acids within the liver—an effect that would likely improve digestion of fat. Cilantro can be helpful in the elimination of heavy metals such as lead, cadmium, arsenic, mercury, and aluminum.

Coriander seeds and cilantro are used extensively in Asian, Latin American, and Spanish foods. The flavor of coriander seeds and leaves combines nicely with beets, onions, potatoes, and lentils. Cilantro is mixed into grain, bean, and meat dishes and used as a garnish.

Using Cilantro and Coriander

- Cilantro leaves can be used in place of basil to make cilantro pesto.

- To make cilantro chutney, combine 1 bunch chopped fresh cilantro, ½ cup shredded coconut, 2 tablespoons chopped fresh mint, and ½ to 1 diced jalapeño pepper.

- Sprinkle ¼ teaspoon ground coriander and ½ teaspoon ground cinnamon in a cup of decaffeinated black tea.

- Heat 1 to 2 tablespoons olive oil, sauté leaves from 1 bunch cleaned spinach, 1 to 2 minced garlic cloves, and 1 to 2 teaspoons coriander seeds. Stir in 1 cup rinsed and drained garbanzo beans and season with ¼ teaspoon ground ginger and ½ teaspoon ground cumin.

- Add ½ teaspoon ground coriander to pancake and waffle batters.

Dill

Dill (*Anethum graveolens*) is a member of the Umbelliferae plant family, along with carrot, celery, fennel, and parsley. Dill is used to calm the stomach and intestines and to counteract sleeplessness. Dill's green leaves are wispy and fernlike and have a soft, sweet taste; both its leaves and seeds flavor food. Dried dill seeds are light brown, winged, and oval with one flat side and two ridges. The leaves and stalks are aromatic and are used fresh or for pickling.

Health Benefits
Like many other herbs, dill's prime health benefit is as a carminative in the elimination of flatulence and digestive disturbances. Like other aromatic herbs, dill has shown some anticancer and antimicrobial effects. It is especially useful in helping the liver get rid of toxic chemicals.

Using Dill

- To make a dill sauce to spoon over cooked potatoes and other vegetables, puree 3 tablespoons extra-virgin olive oil, 2 sprigs dill, 1 teaspoon dill seed, 1 sprig parsley, 1 garlic clove, and the juice and rind of
1 lemon in a blender.

- Combine ¼ cup chopped fresh dill with 1 cup plain yogurt and 1 cup
chopped cucumber for a vegetable dip or as a sauce to serve with grilled
fish and chicken.

- Top fish, especially salmon and trout, with 2 to 3 sprigs dill before
cooking.

- Add 2 teaspoons chopped fresh dill to egg salad.

- Mix 2 cups diced cooked potatoes, 1 cup green beans, and 1 cup
plain yogurt, then season with 2 teaspoons dill seed and 1 tablespoon
chopped fresh dill.

Tarragon

Tarragon (*Artemisia dracunculus*) is a sweet, aromatic herb with a slight peppery flavor reminiscent of fennel, anise, and licorice.

Health Benefits

The traditional medicinal uses of tarragon reflect the high content of active
volatile compounds in its essential oil. Modern research has shown that the
essential oil contains several compounds with potent antimicrobial activity.
When evaluated for its ability to disarm free radicals, tarragon has been found
to have remarkably high antioxidant and free radical–scavenging activity comparable to that of chemicals used commercially in food preservation. The

researchers recommended tarragon as a potential source of natural antioxidants for the food industry.

When diabetic mice received tarragon as part of their diet for nine days, the animals' desire to overeat and excessive thirst were significantly reduced, plus their loss of body weight was lessened—all of which happened without any significant alterations in plasma glucose or insulin concentrations, suggesting that tarragon's beneficial actions occur independently of any improvement of blood sugar control.

Using Tarragon

- Use fresh tarragon to flavor salads, vegetables, and fish.

- Tarragon complements cooked vegetables, such as potatoes, peas, asparagus, carrots, mushrooms, tomatoes, broccoli, and cauliflower. Whisk 1 tablespoon chopped fresh tarragon into 2 eggs before scrambling or making an omelet.

The Magic of Seasonings

Garlic

Garlic, a member of the lily family, is cultivated worldwide and valued not only for its culinary properties but also for its medicinal uses.

Health Benefits

Much of garlic's therapeutic effect is thought to result from its volatile factors, composed of sulfur-containing compounds: allicin, diallyl disulfide, diallyl trisulfide, and others. Other constituents of garlic include additional sulfur-containing compounds, high concentrations of trace minerals (particularly selenium and germanium), glucosinolates, and enzymes. The compound allicin is mainly responsible for the pungent odor of garlic.

The beneficial effects of garlic have been known for thousands of years. Its use as a food should be encouraged, especially in people dealing with elevated cholesterol levels, heart disease, high blood pressure, diabetes, candida infections, asthma, other infections (particularly respiratory tract infections), and gastrointestinal complaints.

Many studies have found that garlic decreases total serum cholesterol levels while increasing serum HDL cholesterol levels. HDL cholesterol, often termed "good" cholesterol, is a protective factor against heart disease. One of the most interesting studies showing the health benefits of garlic was a 1979 study in three populations of vegetarians in the Jain community in India who consumed differing amounts of garlic and onions. The study was significant because the subjects had nearly identical diets, except for their garlic and onion ingestion. Numerous favorable effects on blood lipids were observed in the group that consumed the largest amounts.

Garlic has also demonstrated blood pressure–lowering action, typically decreasing the systolic pressure by 8 mm Hg and the diastolic by 5 mm Hg in patients with high blood pressure. Garlic consumption has also been found to:

- Lower blood sugar levels in diabetics
- Help eliminate heavy metals, such as lead
- Promote detoxification reactions
- Enhance the immune system
- Exert antimicrobial effects

For medicinal purposes, eating at least three cloves of garlic a day is recommended; for general health, an average of four cloves per week is healthful.

Using Garlic

- Buy fresh garlic that is plump and firm. Avoid garlic heads that are soft, show evidence of decay, such as mildew or darkening, or are beginning to sprout.

- When juicing garlic, remove the garlic clove from the bulb and wrap it in some green vegetable leaves, such as parsley or kale. This will keep the garlic from popping out of the juicer, and the chlorophyll from the green leaves will help eliminate some of the odor. Juice the garlic in the leaves first, as the other vegetables will remove the odor from the machine.

- Puree fresh garlic, a can of rinsed and drained garbanzo beans, sesame butter, extra-virgin olive oil, and lemon juice to make a quick dip.

- Sauté leafy, dark green vegetables, such as spinach, kale, and Swiss chard, in 1 tablespoon extra-virgin olive oil and some minced garlic for a quick side dish.

- Wrap a head of garlic in aluminum foil and roast at 350°F for 25 to 30 minutes, or until the garlic can be pierced with a knife. Press each garlic clove to express the softened garlic.

- Mash roasted garlic with boiled or steamed potatoes and some extra-virgin olive oil to make garlic mashed potatoes. Season to taste with pepper and salt substitute.

Ginger

Ginger, with its thick tuberous rhizomes, is a culinary and medicinal power-house. It is native to southeastern Asia, India, and China. You can grow it as a houseplant. It is available in several forms:

- *Whole roots* provide the freshest taste and probably the greatest health benefits. The roots are harvested and shipped while they are still imma-ture and the outer skin is a light green-beige color. Buy plump pieces that are not dried out or moldy.

- *Dried roots* are sold either "black," with the skin left on, or "white," with the skin removed. The dried root is available whole or sliced.

- *Ground ginger* is the ground spice made from dried root.

- *Crystallized ginger* is fresh ginger cooked in sugar syrup, then air-dried and rolled in more sugar.

- *Pickled ginger* is the root sliced paper-thin and pickled in a vinegar solution. This pickle is known in Japan as *gari* and often accompanies sushi.

Health Benefits

More than one hundred clinical studies have been conducted with various forms of ginger. Ginger exerts so many health benefits that it is essential to add it to your diet.

Ginger has a long tradition of alleviating symptoms of gastrointestinal distress. In herbal medicine, ginger is regarded as an excellent carminative (relieves intestinal gas) and intestinal spasmolytic (relaxes and soothes intestinal spasms). These properties can be attributed to its volatile component. In addition to its carminative and intestinal spasmolytic effects, ginger has antioxidant benefits, an ability to inhibit the formation of inflammatory compounds, and direct anti-inflammatory effects. Here is an abridged discussion of some of the key uses.

- Nausea, vomiting, and motion sickness. In one study ginger was shown to be far superior to Dramamine (dimenhydrinate), a commonly used over-the-counter and prescription drug for motion sickness. It can reduce all symptoms associated with motion sickness, including dizziness, nausea, vomiting, and cold sweats. Unlike dimenhydrinate, which works on the central nervous system, ginger affects the gastrointestinal tract and slows the feedback interaction between the stomach and the nausea center in the brain by absorbing and neutralizing gastrointestinal hormones, toxins, and acids. For simple nausea, a cup of ginger tea or a shot of ginger juice may be all you need to settle your stomach.

• Morning sickness. Ginger has been used to treat the nausea and vomiting associated with pregnancy, showing positive results in hyperemesis gravidarum, the most severe form. This condition usually requires
hospitalization. In a double-blind trial, when a dose of 250 mg of ginger powder was administered four times a day, there was a significant
reduction in both the severity of the nausea and the number of vomiting
attacks in nineteen of twenty-seven cases of hyperemesis gravidarum
during early pregnancy (less than twenty weeks).

• Arthritis and inflammation. Ginger contains potent anti-inflammatory
compounds called gingerols that are believed to explain why so many
people with osteoarthritis or rheumatoid arthritis experience a reduction in their pain level and improvement in their mobility when they regularly consume ginger. Gingerols inhibit the formation of inflammatory
cytokines, chemical messengers of the immune system. In one study,
twenty-eight patients with rheumatoid arthritis, eighteen with osteoarthritis, and ten with muscular discomfort were evaluated. Based on clinical
observations, the researchers reported that 75% of the arthritis patients
and 100% of the patients with muscular discomfort experienced relief in
pain or swelling. The recommended dosage was 500 to 1,000 mg per
day, but many patients took three to four times that amount. Patients taking the higher dosages reported quicker and better relief.

• Migraine headaches. The drug sumatriptan (Imitrex) is regarded as the
gold-standard treatment for migraine headaches. It brings about almost
immediate relief for many patients, but headaches recur in almost 40%
of people within twenty-four hours after taking the drug. Minor side
effects of triptans include nausea, dizziness, drowsiness, and muscle
weakness. These medications can also cause more serious side effects,
such as coronary artery spasms, heart attacks, stroke, abnormal heart-
beat, and seizures. In one study, a team of neurologists compared the
effects of ground ginger (250 mg) and sumatriptan (50 mg) in one
hundred men and women who had suffered migraines for an average

of seven years. Results showed that ginger was equally as effective as sumatriptan, achieving 90% relief within two hours after ingestion. Though a small percentage (4%) of those taking ginger experienced minor digestive symptoms, 20% of those taking sumatriptan reported dizziness, drowsiness, or heartburn.

• Excessive menstrual bleeding. Menorrhagia may be prevented by taking ginger. One biochemical abnormality commonly found in the lining of the uterus in women with menorrhagia is an alteration in arachidonic acid metabolism. This fatty acid is derived from meat and dairy sources and is converted to hormonelike compounds known as prostaglandins. The uterine lining of women who have menorrhagia concentrates arachidonic acid to a much greater extent than normal. The increased arachidonic acid release during menstruation results in increased production of a hormonelike compound known as prostaglandin E2 (PGE2), which leads to not only excessive bleeding but also menstrual cramps. Since ginger has been shown to block PGE2 production, researchers assessed the effects of ginger on heavy menstrual bleeding (HMB) in ninety-two young women 15 to 18 years of age. The women took either a 250 mg dried ginger capsule or a placebo capsule three times daily for four consecutive days starting the day before menstrual bleeding commenced. They were followed for three additional consecutive menstrual cycles. During the three intervention cycles, the level of menstrual blood loss of those taking ginger dramatically declined, by 46%, while that of the placebo group dropped by only 2%. The researchers concluded, "Ginger may be considered as an effective therapeutic option for HMB."

Although most scientific studies have used ground ginger root, my feeling is that fresh ginger root at an equivalent dosage will yield even better results because it contains active enzymes. Though some studies have shown positive results with dosages as low as 250 mg of ground ginger root, most of the studies utilized 1 gram, equivalent to approximately 10 grams or ⅓ ounce of fresh ginger root, roughly a ¼-inch slice.

Using Ginger

Whenever possible, choose fresh ginger over dried since it is not only superior in flavor but also contains higher levels of anti-inflammatory compounds. Fresh ginger can be purchased in the produce section at supermarkets. The bronze root should show no signs of decay such as soft spots, mildew, or a dry, wrinkled skin.

- Taking a daily shot of fresh, raw ginger juice is one of the best ways to take advantage of this healing food. I recommend eating or drinking fresh ginger if you have rheumatoid arthritis, migraine headaches, or any other inflammatory condition. There are endless ways to use ginger as a spice. Ginger is also available as a supplement.

- A piece of fresh ginger adds zip to any fresh juice or smoothie.

- Make your own ginger ale. It is a super replacement for sugary soft drinks. It is also useful in relieving intestinal upset. Juice a ½- to 1-inch slice of ginger, 1 lemon wedge with peel, and 1 Granny Smith apple, cut into wedges. Juice the ginger first, then the lemon wedge and apple. Pour the juice into a glass, and stir in 4 ounces sparkling mineral water.

- Ginger tea is fantastic when you feel a cold coming on. It is a diaphoretic tea, meaning that it will warm you from the inside and promote perspiration. It's also good when you don't have a cold and just want to warm up and feel good! To make ginger tea: If you have a juice extractor, juice a 1-inch piece of ginger and ¼ lemon and add the mixture to 1 cup hot water. Or mince the ginger and steep in the hot water with the lemon wedge. For an additional flavor boost, add ⅛ teaspoon grated nutmeg or ground cardamom.

- For a gingery salad dressing, whisk together 4 tablespoons sesame oil, 2 tablespoons rice vinegar, 1 tablespoon tamari, ½ teaspoon grated fresh ginger, and 1 mashed garlic clove (optional).

- For stir-fried vegetable dishes, add 1 teaspoon grated fresh ginger for each cup of vegetables while cooking. The strength of the taste that ginger imparts to a dish depends on when it is added during the cooking process. If it is added at the beginning, it will lend a subtler taste; it will be much more pungent if stirred in at the end.

Horseradish

Horseradish (*Armoracia rusticana* and *Armoracia lapathifolia*) is a long, tapered root with a thin, light brown skin, white flesh, and spiky green leaves. It is a member of the cabbage family.

Although the leaves can be used in salads, horseradish is valued primarily for its root's pungent bite. This effect, which develops only when the root is broken and wet, is the result of the reaction that occurs when a number of chemicals that the plant stores separately are allowed to mingle.

Health Benefits

The medicinal properties of horseradish are underresearched. It is known that horseradish definitely helps protect against food-borne illnesses. Recent research shows that horseradish protects against *Listeria*, *E. coli*, *Staphylococcus aureus*, and other food pathogens. The reason is allylisothiocyanate, one of the pungent chemicals formed when horseradish is cut. This powerful antibacterial ingredient constitutes 60% of horseradish oil.

Horseradish is also a cholagogue, an agent that stimulates the release of bile from the gallbladder. It can help maintain a healthy gallbladder and improve digestion. Increasing bile secretion is a part of digesting dietary fats and oils as well as secreting cholesterol and waste from the body.

Using Horseradish

- Toss 2 cups roasted and diced beets with ½ cup extra-virgin olive oil and 3 tablespoons balsamic vinegar. Add 1 teaspoon coarse salt, ½ teaspoon freshly ground black pepper, 1 cup chopped red onions, ¼ cup plain nonfat yogurt, and ⅓ cup freshly grated horseradish. Mix well before serving.

- For cranberry-horseradish sauce, in a saucepan combine ¾ cup boiling water, ½ cup honey, and ½ cup brown sugar and stir until dissolved. Add 1 (10-ounce) package of fresh cranberries, return to a boil, and cook for 10 minutes. Cool slightly and stir in 2 tablespoons freshly grated horseradish and 1 tablespoon Dijon mustard. Chill before serving.

- For a sauce to accompany fish or shrimp, whisk together 1 cup orange marmalade, 3 tablespoons Dijon mustard, and 1 tablespoon freshly grated horseradish.

- Stir 1½ teaspoons to 1 tablespoon horseradish into soups when serving.

- Whisk 1 tablespoon prepared horseradish into ½ cup salad dressing.

- Mix a spoonful of horseradish with ½ cup plain nonfat yogurt, 4 tablespoons butter, and ½ teaspoon Dijon mustard. Add to corn on the cob, cooked carrots, green beans, peas, or new potatoes for a flavor boost.

Salt

Salt is a mineral that is essential to human health but should be consumed in proper quantities. Too much sodium in the diet from salt (sodium chloride) can disrupt this balance. Many people know that a high-sodium, low-potassium diet can cause high blood pressure, while the opposite can dangerously lower blood pressure. Most people don't realize that consumption of too much salt also raises the risk of cancer, heart disease, and diabetes.

Salts used in food are mined from the earth or evaporated from seawater. Salt brings out the flavors of many foods, but it's important not to use too much. If you must use salt, I suggest trying one of the salt substitutes made of potassium chloride, such as AlsoSalt, LoSalt, Nu-Salt, and NoSalt. Though potassium chloride possesses some of the salty characteristics of sodium chloride, it also has a somewhat bitter metallic aftertaste that some people do not like. However, there are some better forms of salt substitutes on the market that provide a saltiness and mouthfeel that are close to sodium chloride. Some mix potassium chloride with sodium chloride to cut the sodium in half; just be aware that they still contain salt.

The World Health Organization recommends limiting sodium intake to less than 2,000 mg per day, and the American Heart Association recommends limiting it to less than 1,500 mg per day. My recommendation is to go even lower, to less than 1,000 mg per day. That recommendation is particularly important to the eighty million Americans with high blood pressure.

In the United States, only 5% of sodium intake comes from the natural ingredients in food. Prepared foods contribute 45% of our sodium intake, 45% is added in cooking, and another 5% is added as a condiment. You can reduce your salt intake by following these tips:

- Remove the saltshaker from the table.

- Omit added salt when preparing food. Read food labels carefully to determine the amounts of sodium they contain. Learn to recognize ingredients that contain sodium. Salt, soy sauce, salt brine, and any ingredient including "sodium" (such as monosodium glutamate) or "baking soda" (sodium bicarbonate) as part of its name contains sodium.

- When reading labels and menus, look for words that signal high sodium content, such as smoked, barbecued, pickled, broth, soy sauce, teriyaki, marinated, cocktail sauce, tomato base, and Parmesan.

- Avoid canned vegetables and soups, which are often high in sodium, even the low-sodium versions.

Using Salt

- Learn to enjoy the flavors of unsalted foods.
- Use herbs, spices, garlic, ginger, vinegar, lemon juice, and other flavorings in your cooking.
- When dining out, ask the server to tell the chef that you want your food unsalted.

Sugar and Sweeteners

The research is now overwhelming and beyond debate: excessive consumption of sugar, high-fructose corn syrup, and other refined sugars is a major contributing factor in a wide variety of diseases and premature aging. Sugar is the new cigarette in terms of public health hazard.

Eating too much sugar can be harmful to blood sugar control and is associated with increased risk for obesity, heart disease, and some forms of cancer. Currently, more than half of the carbohydrates consumed in the United States are in the form of sugars being added to foods as sweetening agents.

The consumption of sweeteners in the United States increased from about fourteen million tons in 1979 to about twenty-two million tons in 1999. Let me break that down into practical terms. In the 1970s, the typical American consumed approximately 27 teaspoons of added sugar per person per day, but by 2000 that amount increased to more than 33 teaspoons per person per day. Not surprisingly, it was during this period that the US population saw the biggest jump in obesity and diabetes. The consumption of sugar-sweetened beverages has played the largest role in the increase of added sweeteners in the American diet. Food consumption studies have found that the recent increases in energy intake coincide with increased consumption of soft drinks.

What is staggering is that the intake of synthetic noncaloric sweeteners such as aspartame and sucralose also seems to contribute to diabetes and obesity (discussed below).

The increase in sugar intake over the past forty years has been due primarily to the increase in the use of high-fructose corn syrup (HFCS). In spite of its name, there is no more fructose in high-fructose corn syrup than there is sucrose. HFCS is simply sweet and is much less expensive than sucrose. Many different products use HFCS as an ingredient, including beverages, cereals, baked goods, dairy products, candy, and many other processed foods. More than 5% of the total American corn crop goes to making HFCS.

Artificial Sweeteners

The common belief that consumption of artificial sweeteners such as aspartame, sucralose, and saccharin will lead to a reduction in the number of calories consumed and weight loss has repeatedly been shown to be false. In fact, some studies have shown that artificial sweeteners may actually increase appetite.

Another line of research shows that artificial sweeteners can actually create insulin resistance via alterations in the gut microbiome. This effect has been shown in both mice and humans. Think about it: many people who are overweight, obese, or living with type 2 diabetes reach for diet drinks and other artificially sweetened foods and beverages, thinking they will help their blood sugar control. In actuality, artificial sweeteners add fuel to the fire.

Artificial sweeteners also increase the risk of depression. A study conducted by researchers at the National Institutes of Health (NIH) showed that adults who drank artificially sweetened beverages—diet drinks in particular—were 30% more likely to develop depression than those who did not drink such beverages. The study was huge, as it involved 263,925 people between ages 50 and 71 years at enrollment. The risk of depression was greatest among those who drank more than 32 ounces per day of diet soda or other diet beverages. Drinking 32 ounces per day of regular soda or sweetened beverages was also associated with a greater risk of depression.

Instead of drinking beverages containing artificial sweeteners or a lot of sugar, look to nature for low-calorie sweeteners. These are available in both liquid and solid (powder or granulated) forms. Use them on an as-needed basis as substitutes for sugar and artificial sweeteners. Your choices include:

- Stevia is a natural sweetener extracted from the *Stevia rebaudiana* plant. Some stevia compounds are 300 times as sweet as sugar, and stevia has an excellent safety profile.

- Monk fruit or luo han guo extract is not as popular as stevia, but it may actually be a little sweeter, without the bitter aftertaste.

- Sugar alcohols or polyol sweeteners such as erythritol, xylitol, sorbitol, mannitol, and maltitol are safe in moderate dosages. Because they are poorly absorbed at higher dosages—more than 10 grams daily—they can cause gastrointestinal upset ranging from mild discomfort to severe diarrhea, especially in children because of their smaller size.

- Allulose, the newest member of the natural sweetener family, is a naturally occurring sugar that is produced from corn via an enzymatic reaction. It is nearly as sweet as sugar, but has only one-tenth the calorie count of sucrose or fructose. It is absorbed from the gastrointestinal tract, so it does not cause the GI side effects of the polyols. But it is not utilized by the body as an energy source, so it is excreted in the urine. It holds much promise as a direct replacement for sugar in many products including baked goods, beverages, and other foods. It also helps insulin work better and may be the perfect sugar to promote weight loss.

- Tagatose is a natural sugar found in apples, pineapples, oranges, raisins, whole wheat, and milk. It is a low-calorie sweetener that is 92% as sweet as sugar and has the same look, feel, and bulk. It is only now becoming more popular as a bulk sweetener combined with stevia and monk fruit extract. It is also just emerging as a sweetener in a variety of different products in health food stores, from nutritional bars to protein powders and chocolates. Tagatose acts more like a form of fiber than a sugar. As a result, it provides significant health benefits, including a favorable effect on the gut microbiome. Perhaps the biggest health benefit is that tagatose, like allulose, actually helps promote weight loss.

———————————

Using more spices, herbs, and other seasonings in food helps fight diseases and wakes up your palate. Once you start adding more flavors to your food, you'll find that you'll want to amp up the taste even more. This is nature's way of encouraging us to take advantage of the magical effects that herbs, spices, and other seasonings can have on our bodies.

8

The Synergetic Diet with Recipes

The Synergetic Diet incorporates the best foods from the most healthful diets studied by scientists and researchers from around the world. When my patients ask me what they should eat to deal with certain conditions and enjoy a healthy lifestyle, this is the advice I give.

Synergetic Diet Pyramid

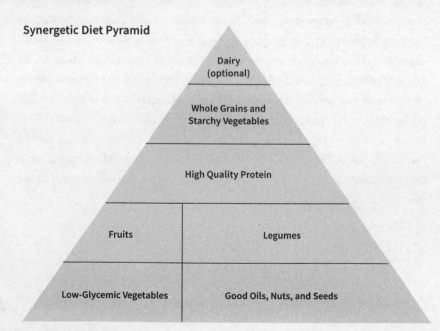

Eat a Variety of Foods

As previously mentioned, people who eat a variety of different foods have a lower rate of obesity than people who consume the same foods daily and weekly. Most Americans repeatedly eat the same foods, making for a monotonous diet. It's possible that many people's excessive calorie and food consumption may be some sort of physiological craving gone awry. Perhaps the brain is seeking to help improve the body's nutritional intake by sending signals to eat, but somehow it is just causing excessive cravings for additional calories in general instead of giving the brain the specific nutrients it needs to feel satisfied. Despite this possibility, there is not a lot of research in this area. There are numerous case histories in the medical literature of people having specific food cravings, indicating some sort of physiological basis for them. For example, eating of dirt or chewing ice cubes is often an indication of iron deficiency. Research done by the US Army showed that when well-nourished men were placed on monotonous diets, it led to increased craving for foods that were not provided. But there is little research into whether individuals who habitually consume a monotonous diet are more likely to consume more calories than those eating a more varied diet. Remember earlier in chapter 2, I mentioned a study by researchers at the Harvard School of Public Health and New York University School of Medicine showed that greater dietary variety is inversely associated with obesity. The greater the variety of healthful food, the greater the protection against excess body weight. A varied diet makes our food choices more interesting and less boring. Eating the same foods and menus again and again is a sure path to food boredom. Dietary variety wakes up the senses and makes eating more interesting and fun. Again, one of my goals in writing this book is to instill the importance of eating a broader spectrum of health-promoting foods. Take advantage of all the wonderful foods that you have access to.

Focus on Raw Fruits and Vegetables

A simple, effective method to help promote weight loss is to focus on raw fruits and vegetables. Detailed clinical studies have shown that diets containing a high percentage (up to 60% of calories) of uncooked foods are associated with significant weight loss and lowering of blood pressure in overweight individuals. Raw-food diets produce these effects in the following ways:

- A raw-food diet provides higher levels of many nutrients. Cooking can cause the loss of up to 97% of water-soluble vitamins (B vitamins and vitamin C) and up to 40% of the fat-soluble vitamins (A, D, E, and K). Since uncooked foods most often contain more vitamins and other nutrients, they may help increase the feeling of satisfaction from food, leading to a reduced calorie intake.

- The blood pressure–lowering effect of raw foods is most likely due to their fiber and potassium content. When patients are switched from a raw-food diet to a cooked-food diet (without a change in calorie or sodium content), there is a rapid increase in blood pressure, back to the prestudy levels.

- A diet in which an average of 60% of the calories ingested comes from raw foods reduces stress on the body. Specifically, the presence of enzymes in raw foods, the reduced allergenic effects of raw foods, and the effects of raw foods on our gut bacterial flora are thought to aid digestion, compared to a diet focused on cooked foods.

Juice Your Fruits and Vegetables

It would take you a long time to sit down and eat all the fresh fruits and vegetables that are necessary to reach the goal of ingesting 60% of total calories from raw, uncooked foods. Juicing those fruits and vegetables is a quick and easy way to get the nutrition you need. As a bonus, fresh juice helps the body's digestive process and enables quick absorption of high-quality nutrition, resulting in increased energy levels. This effect is one of the greatest advantages of utilizing fresh juice in a weight-loss plan.

One of the most common questions that I get when I talk about the wonders of fresh fruit and vegetable juice is "Why juice? Aren't we supposed to eat whole fruits and vegetables to get the fiber?" The answer: of course you are, but you should drink fresh juice, too. Juicing quickly provides the most easily digestible and concentrated nutritional benefits of fruits and vegetables.

Fresh juices are far superior to canned, bottled, or frozen juices, because they contain enzymes and other "living" ingredients. Canned, bottled, and packaged juices have been pasteurized, which makes them shelf stable but causes the loss of nutrients such as vitamins and minerals.

To illustrate this, a group of researchers at Health Canada designed a study comparing the antiviral activity of fresh apple juice to commercial apple juice from concentrate, apple cider, and apple wine. The most potent antiviral activity was found in fresh apple juice. Why? Commercial apple juices are produced using methods such as pasteurization that destroy enzymes and alter many key compounds. In doing so, a great deal of the antiviral activity is also lost. Furthermore, although the fresh juice was greatly superior in health benefits to the other products, it lost its potency during storage, so you should drink juice as soon as it's made. The compounds that are thought to be responsible for the antiviral activity are various flavonoid molecules, which are found in highest quantities in fresh apple juice.

Fresh apple juice also contains ellagic acid, a compound that exerts potent antioxidant and anticancer effects. Ellagic acid protects against damage to the chromosomes and blocks the cancer-causing actions of many pollutants, such as polycyclic aromatic hydrocarbons (PAH), found in cigarette smoke, and toxic chemicals such as benzopyrene. Ellagic acid is not destroyed by freezing or freeze-drying, but it can be destroyed by heat. Whereas fresh whole apples and fresh apple juice contain approximately 100 to 130 mg of ellagic acid per 100 grams (roughly 3½ ounces), the amount found in cooked or commercial apple products is at or near zero. The flavonoid and ellagic acid content is high in many berries, particularly raspberries and blackberries, which can contain up to 1.5 mg of ellagic acid per gram.

Another example of how freshness impacts nutritional value is dietary glutathione. Glutathione is a small protein composed of three amino acids that are manufactured in cells, but sometimes we don't make enough of it to keep up with the demand. Glutathione is not only the most important antioxidant in the body, it also aids in the detoxification of heavy metals such as lead and in the elimination of pesticides and solvents. When researchers measured the glutathione levels in foods, they found that fresh fruits and vegetables provide excellent levels of glutathione but processed ones do not—more evidence showing that the greatest benefit from our foods comes from fresh ones.

Best Juices for Weight Loss

Some juices are better than others for promoting weight loss. The most effective are those that are dense in nutrients but low in calories. The first five vegetables listed below are not only nutrient dense, they are also quite strongly flavored. Mixing them with carrot, apple, or tomato juice will make them more palatable. Notice that the fruits are farther down on the scale than the vegetables. Although fruits are full of valuable nutrients, they contain more natural sugars than vegetables. This means they are higher in calories and also have the potential to stress blood sugar control, so they should be used sparingly (no more than two servings of whole fruit or in juice form per day). When juicing, add some fresh, peeled ginger or half a lemon to the juicer to add some zing and kick up both your AMPk activity and your metabolism. Here in descending order are the most nutrient-dense fruits and vegetables suitable for juicing.

- Bell peppers
- Parsley
- Kale
- Broccoli
- Spinach
- Celery
- Carrots
- Cabbage
- Beets
- Lemons
- Pineapple
- Cantaloupe
- Watermelon
- Tomatoes
- Apples
- Strawberries
- Pears

Drink Water to Lose Weight and Stay Healthy

Water is essential to life. It is necessary to replace the water that is lost through urination, sweat, and breathing. Even mild dehydration impairs physiologic and performance responses.

Many nutrients dissolve in water and thus can be absorbed more easily by the digestive tract. Similarly, many metabolic processes need to occur in water. Water is a component of blood and thus is important for transporting chemicals and nutrients to cells and tissues. Each cell is constantly bathed in a watery fluid. Water also carries waste materials from cells to the kidneys for filtering and elimination. Water absorbs and transports heat. For example, heat produced by muscle cells during exercise is carried by water in the blood to the body surface, helping to maintain the right temperature balance. The skin cells also release water as perspiration, which helps maintain body temperature.

Several factors are thought to increase the likelihood of chronic mild dehydration: a faulty thirst "alarm" in the brain; dissatisfaction with the taste of water; regular exercise that increases the amount of water lost through sweat; living in a hot, dry climate; and consumption of the natural diuretics caffeine and alcohol.

Drinking water before a meal can acutely reduce caloric intake during the meal, especially among middle-aged and older adults. In one study, forty-eight overweight adults aged 55 to 75 years were assigned to one of two groups: (1) a low-calorie diet plus 500 ml water prior to each daily meal (water group) or (2) a low-calorie diet alone (nonwater group). Weight loss was approximately 4 pounds greater in the water-drinking group than in the non-water-drinking group. The water-drinking group showed a 44% greater decline in weight over the twelve weeks than did the non-water-drinking group. Thus, when combined with a low-calorie diet, consuming 500 ml water prior to each main meal led to greater weight loss than a low-calorie diet alone in middle-aged and older adults.

There is currently a great deal of concern over the purity of the US water supply. Most of the water supply is full of chemicals, including routinely added chlorine, as well as toxic organic compounds and chemicals, such as PCBs, pesticide residues, and nitrates, and heavy metals such as lead, mercury, and cadmium. It is estimated that lead alone may contaminate the water of more than forty million Americans. You can determine the safety of your tap or well water by asking your local water company to perform a routine analysis.

If you drink bottled water, be aware that although bottles these days are made from BPA-free plastic, they are laced with other chemicals that can leach into the water if the bottles are exposed to heat or sit around for a long time.

Four Ways to Drink More Water

- Set a specific goal of how much water you want to drink every day. Setting a goal creates awareness. Aim for at least 2 to 3 quarts of water a day.

- Download an app to your smart phone to help you reach your daily water intake goals. Such an app allows you to set reminders to drink water at scheduled or random intervals and keep track of how well you are meeting your daily goals. "Waterlogged" is the most popular app.

- Have a glass of water before every meal and snack, especially if you want to lose weight.

- I find that I drink more water if I add a squeeze of citrus juice. You can also flavor water by adding strawberries, cucumbers, mint, ginger, or watermelon. I also drink a lot of tea, fresh juices, protein shakes, and other healthy beverages that count toward my daily recommended amount.

Use Spices, Herbs, and Seasonings to Rev Up Your Metabolism and Activate AMPk

Chapter 7, "Spice It Up!" is entirely devoted to using spices, herbs, and other seasonings, but this is so important to the Synergetic Diet that I want to reiterate it here. It seems that every culinary herb and spice that has been examined for its effects on AMPk has been found to be an AMPk activator. Some examples tested and shown to have this activity include turmeric, cayenne pepper, ginger, basil, oregano, rosemary, sage, thyme, cinnamon, clove, black pepper, and garlic. The takeaway: adding herbs and spices to your food can help boost your metabolism. Spicy foods may help people lose weight. The principal ingredients in curry, for instance, all contain compounds that activate AMPk. Most of the research on the weight-loss effects of these ingredients has focused on animal studies with impressive results. A few human studies, mainly with cayenne pepper, that focused on its capsaicin content, the compound that gives red pepper its hot and spicy character, have shown that cayenne pepper intake increases the basal metabolic rate while reducing appetite and caloric intake. Moreover, there are other components in red pepper that also seem to help activate fat-burning actions. Get into the habit of liberally adding herbs and spices to your foods.

Organic Versus Conventionally Grown Foods

When people ask me if it's worth it to pay more for organically grown foods, my answer is yes, for the following reasons.

- They reduce your exposure to health-robbing toxins used in conventional agricultural practices, including pesticides, heavy metals such as lead and mercury, and solvents such as benzene and toluene. A number of pesticides have already been recognized as carcinogens, while others have been shown to negatively affect mitochondrial energy production. Still others damage cellular membranes, triggering inflammation that has been linked to atherosclerosis. Heavy metals lower IQ and damage nerve function, contributing to neurodegenerative diseases such as Parkinson's disease, Alzheimer's disease, and multiple sclerosis. Solvents damage white blood cells, the immune system defenders that enable the body to resist infections. Not only are these toxic substances individually harmful, but when combined and used in commercially grown and processed foods, their effects in the human body, where they accumulate, have been found to be magnified as much as a thousandfold.

- They increase your consumption of health-promoting micronutrients. A number of studies have demonstrated that organically grown produce contains significantly higher amounts of many vitamins and minerals. In a 1988 review of thirty-four studies that compared organic with conventionally grown foods, organic food was found to have higher protein quality in all comparisons, higher levels of vitamin C in 58% of all studies, and 5% to 20% higher mineral levels for all but two minerals. In some cases, the mineral levels in organically grown foods were dramatically higher—as much as three times as high in one study involving iron content. Organically grown foods also contain higher amounts of plant protective compounds such as flavonoids and carotenoids. Take resveratrol, for example, a compound produced by grapes in self-defense against environmental stressors such as attacks by insects or fungal infection. Organically grown grapes produce much higher amounts of resveratrol than do conventionally grown grapes, which are protected by treatment with man-made fungicides.

- They safeguard your children's health. Reports from the Natural Resources Defense Council and the Environmental Working Group (EWG) have found that millions of American children are exposed to levels of pesticides in their food that surpass limits considered safe. Some of these pesticides are known neurotoxins with the potential to harm a developing brain and nervous system. Others, with carcinogenic activity, may wreak even more damage in children and adolescents, whose higher growth rates involve higher rates of cell turnover, particularly as their sexual organs develop.

- They safeguard the health of the environment. Residues from toxic chemicals used in conventional farming methods remain in the soil and leach into groundwater. According to the Environmental Protection Agency, pesticides (some known to be carcinogens) now pollute the groundwater—the primary source of drinking water—in thirty-eight states, where more than half the country's population lives. The use of chemical-dependent farming methods has not only adversely impacted soil and water but also reduced biodiversity, as well as the nutrient quality and taste of our foods, since synthetic nitrate fertilizers cause nitrate to bind to water, which makes the produce look good but lessens its flavor. Organic farming practices work to preserve and protect the environment by maintaining a restorative and sustainable biosystem, which improves soil quality, preserves water purity, encourages biodiversity, and, by nourishing the soil, produces plants that are rich in flavor as well as nutrients.

The Dirty Dozen and Consistently Clean Fifteen

The Environmental Working Group is a nonprofit consumer advocacy group composed of scientists, engineers, policy experts, lawyers, and computer programmers who work together to expose threats to our health and the environment and to find solutions to them. Each year this organization puts together "The Shopper's Guide to Pesticides in Produce" and boils its findings into two popular lists:

Most Contaminated: The Dirty Dozen

Because of the high levels of fertilizers and pesticides found in these foods when conventionally grown, buy organic ones whenever possible.

Strawberries	Tomatoes
Apples	Sweet bell peppers
Nectarines	Cherry tomatoes
Peaches	Cucumbers
Celery	Hot peppers
Grapes	Kale
Cherries	Collard greens
Spinach	

Least Contaminated: The Clean Fifteen

The following foods are the least contaminated of all conventionally grown food, but it is still best to purchase organic varieties whenever possible.

Avocados	Papayas
Sweet corn	Kiwifruit
Pineapples	Eggplant
Cabbage	Honeydew melon
Peas	Grapefruit
Onions	Cantaloupe
Asparagus	Cauliflower
Mangoes	

Daily Meal Plan and Synergetic Diet Recipes

Here is a simple template for a daily menu plan. Pages 206–209 provide a four-day menu plan as an example of how to use the template.

Breakfast
Focus on high-protein foods and smoothies to start the day.

Midmorning Snack
A 100- to 150-calorie snack focusing on low-glycemic, high-fiber, and high-water-content (volumetric) foods.

Lunch
A low-glycemic, high-volumetric lunch. Focus on salads and soups.

Midafternoon Snack
Another 100- to 150-calorie snack focusing on low-glycemic, high-fiber, and high-water-content (volumetric) foods.

Dinner
A low-glycemic, high-protein, high-volumetric meal. One serving (50 to 100 grams) of baked chicken breast, salmon, lean meat, or tofu; a fresh salad dressed with extra-virgin olive oil and natural herbs and spices; one serving (1 to 2 cups) of a cooked nonstarchy vegetable; and ½ cup berries for dessert.

Evening Snack or Tea
A 100- to 150-calorie snack focusing on low-glycemic, high-volumetric foods or, better yet, 1 or 2 cups of herbal tea (no caffeine).

Breakfast

Consuming high-quality protein in the morning is a critical tool in weight loss. Starting the day with a high-protein breakfast can promote prolonged satiety. I drink a smoothie with whey protein or eat one cup of cooked organic egg whites or egg white substitute mixed with one organic whole egg. A smoothie gives me 25 grams of protein on the days I work out, while the eggs provide 50 grams on the days I don't. On the days I work out, I usually eat a protein bar after exercising that provides another 15 to 20 grams of protein. Here are some other suggestions.

Treat eggs like a blank canvas; all kinds of herbs, seasonings, and vegetables can be added to them. Try fresh herbs such as basil, parsley, or dill; spice blends such as curry or chili powder; and chopped vegetables such as broccoli, spinach, and sun-dried tomatoes. Pair the eggs with a side of berries, sliced tomatoes, or a nonstarchy vegetable, such as cooked asparagus.

Mix one cup unsweetened, nonfat plain Greek yogurt with berries or other fresh fruit. Add 2.5 to 5 grams of PGX to the yogurt first if you are trying to lose weight. Eat dinner for breakfast. Try poached salmon, grilled chicken, or scrambled tofu with vegetables.

Here are a few of my favorite smoothie recipes. I prefer whey protein, but you can substitute a vegetarian/vegan protein source (pea, soy, rice, hemp, etc.) if you desire. Puree everything in a blender, pour into a glass, and enjoy.

Apple-Cinnamon Smoothie

8 ounces unsweetened vanilla almond milk, rice milk, or soy milk
25 to 30 grams whey protein
1 small red apple, chopped
¼ to ½ teaspoon ground cinnamon

Berry Smoothie

8 ounces unsweetened vanilla almond milk, rice milk, or soy milk
25 to 30 grams whey protein, any flavor
½ cup fresh strawberries, blueberries, or raspberries or a combination

Vanilla Ice Smoothie

8 ounces unsweetened vanilla almond milk, rice milk, or soy milk
25 to 30 grams vanilla whey protein
½ teaspoon pure vanilla extract
3 to 4 ice cubes

Healthy Oatmeal

Though many people eat cereals in the morning, know that they set your body up for straining your blood sugar control later in the day. If you are going to eat oatmeal or another whole grain cereal, add some PGX to reduce the glycemic load. Though I occasionally eat this for breakfast, I often enjoy it as a late-evening snack.

1 serving

⅓ cup instant oatmeal
10 grams vanilla or unflavored whey protein
1 to 2 tablespoons xylitol or natural stevia-based sweetener, or to taste
2.5 to 5 grams PGX granules
1 teaspoon ground cinnamon

Bring 1½ cups of water to a boil. In a small bowl, mix the oatmeal, whey protein, sweetener, PGX, and cinnamon. Add the boiling water to the bowl and stir vigorously.

Mediterranean Omelet

1 tablespoon extra-virgin olive oil
¼ red bell pepper, seeded and cut into ½-inch pieces
⅛ cup diced onions
½ garlic clove, minced
1 tablespoon minced sun-dried tomatoes packed in oil
⅓ cup egg substitute
1 tablespoon grated mozzarella cheese

Heat a nonstick skillet over medium heat. Add the olive oil, bell pepper, onions, and garlic and sauté until soft. Add the tomatoes, then pour in the egg substitute and rotate the pan to distribute evenly. Lift the edges of the omelet, tilting the pan to allow the liquid to run under the cooked egg substitute. Lower the heat to medium low and cook, without stirring the eggs, until set. On one-half of the omelet, sprinkle the cheese, then fold over the enclosing cheese.

Snacks

In order to meet the desired intake of health-promoting foods, snacking on healthy foods is an absolute must. If you don't have in-between-meal snacks, too much stress is put on your digestive system and physiology. Spread your nutrition and calories throughout the day with balanced meals and snacks rather than loading up on the wrong foods when your hunger and cravings kick in.

When it comes to snacking, keep the portion sizes small and calorie counts low. Cut-up vegetables and fruits, fresh juice, green tea, nuts, and seeds all make for great snacking. On days that I work out, I have a protein bar and a mug of hot cacao brew (see page 102) midmorning. On nonworkout days, I just drink a cup of my special brew.

My Favorite Juice Recipes

Fresh juice also makes for a great midmorning or midafternoon snack. Here are some of my favorites. Each recipe yields 8 to 12 ounces fresh juice. The actual yield will depend on the size of the fruits or vegetables and the kind of juicer used. Unless otherwise noted, all of the recipes call for medium-size fruits and vegetables. I have noted which ones are particularly good for weight loss and detoxification with an asterisk (*).

Better Red Than Dead*

This drink is rich in carotene content, especially the red and orange ones. I call this drink "Better Red Than Dead" because one of my professors, Dr. Ed Madison, once gave a lecture with this title on the benefits of carotenes. His lecture made an impression on me, and I have tried to maintain a high carotene intake ever since. Be sure to scrub and wash the beet and its greens well.

1 beet, including stems and leaves
½ sweet potato, cut into strips
3 carrots

Juice the beet first, then the sweet potato strips, and then the carrots.

Juice Up Your Morning

Pears and apples are excellent sources of water-soluble fibers such as pectin, while plums have laxative properties.

2 pitted plums
2 apples, cut into wedges
1 pear, sliced

Juice the plums, apples, and pear alternately.

....

Color Me Pink*

If you are on a weight-loss program, start the day with this low-calorie, high-in-flavonoids juice. The natural fruit sugars will keep your appetite in check. Leave as much of the white pith under the peel of the grapefruit as possible, as it is rich in flavonoids.

1 cup raspberries
1 large pink grapefruit, peeled

Juice the raspberries first, then the grapefruit.

....

Digestive Delight

A fantastic drink for people who have trouble with indigestion. Packed with enzymes, ginger, and mint, this soothing drink will help ease spastic intestines and promote the elimination of gas.

1-inch slice fresh ginger
½ cup fresh mint leaves
2 kiwifruit, unpeeled
¼ pineapple with skin, sliced lengthwise

Juice the ginger and mint first, followed by the kiwifruit and then the pineapple.

....

Casanova

Ginger has been shown to possess some mild aphrodisiac effects and has a long history of use as a sexual aid in the Arabic system of medicine. The parsley will provide increased energy and awareness.

1-inch slice fresh ginger
Handful of fresh flat-leaf parsley
¼ pineapple with skin, sliced

Place the ginger in the middle of the parsley and feed into the juicer first. Then juice the pineapple.

....

Fennel Citrus Mix*

Fennel combines really well with citrus to make a great breakfast or refreshing drink.

1 small fennel bulb, trimmed
1 large grapefruit
1 orange

Juice the fennel first, followed by the grapefruit and orange.

....

Everything But the Kitchen Sink*

What to do with one apple, three carrots, and other small amounts of vegetables in the refrigerator? If you have two apples and one carrot, no problem. This juice includes the best of everything.

Handful of spinach
2 celery ribs
3 carrots
2 radishes with tops
1 apple, cut into wedges
½ cucumber
1 tomato, quartered
½ cup broccoli florets with stems
½ green bell pepper, seeded

Juice the spinach first, followed by the celery to push it through. Alternate the remaining vegetables, with a carrot coming last.

....

Mint Foam

This great drink is "fun-tasting." Mint has a soothing effect on the intestinal tract and also exhibits some antiviral activity.

Handful of fresh mint
2 kiwifruit, peeled
1 Granny Smith apple, cut into wedges

Juice the mint first, followed by the kiwifruit, then the apple. Pour over ice, if desired.

....

Female Balance*

This drink supports the female glandular system. Both fennel and celery contain phytoestrogens, plant compounds that can occupy binding sites for female hormones and exert hormonelike effects. This drink is helpful in a wide range of conditions specific to women, including menopause and PMS, due to the phytoestrogens and important nutrients (such as potassium, magnesium, folic acid, and vitamin B_6) in the juice.

1 small fennel bulb
1 apple, cut into wedges
4 celery stalks

Cut the fennel into narrow wedges and feed it into the juicer, followed by the apple and celery.

....

Ginger Ale*

This is a great drink for children, a super replacement for sugary soft drinks. It is also useful in relieving intestinal upset.

½-inch slice fresh ginger
1 lemon wedge with peel
1 Granny Smith apple, cut into wedges
4 ounces sparkling mineral water

Juice the ginger first, followed by the lemon wedge, and then the apple. Stir in the mineral water.

....

Go Green Drink*

This is one of the healthiest juice recipes in the book.

Handful of fresh flat-leaf parsley or wheatgrass
1 Granny Smith apple, cut into wedges
2 kale leaves
Handful of spinach
4 celery stalks

Juice the parsley first, then the apple, kale, spinach, and celery.

....

Mike's Favorite

From the name of the recipe, it is obvious that I like this drink. It is thick and filling, and I frequently have it for breakfast.

1-inch slice fresh ginger
1 cup blueberries
¼ pineapple with skin, sliced

Juice the ginger first, then the blueberries, and finally the pineapple.

....

Lunch

Most supermarkets and grocery stores now sell organic mixed greens in the produce section, which makes it convenient and easy to put a salad together. Wash the greens even if the package says they are prewashed. Choose 2 cups chopped of one or a mixture of romaine lettuce, iceberg lettuce, spinach, Boston or Bibb lettuce, endive, arugula, escarole, kale, or watercress. Add 1 cup of a mixture of alfalfa sprouts; fresh berries; diced bell peppers, carrots, and cucumber; torn fresh herbs; sliced mushrooms and radishes; and chopped tomatoes and zucchini. Toss together in a bowl with 1 tablespoon salad dressing.

Synergetic Salad Dressing

Make a jar of this dressing at the beginning of the week and use it throughout the week. Be sure to shake well before using.

24 servings (1¼ cups)

½ cup extra-virgin olive, avocado, or macadamia nut oil
½ cup organic flaxseed oil
2 tablespoons fresh lemon juice
2 tablespoons balsamic vinegar
1 tablespoon dried Italian seasoning
1 teaspoon salt substitute
1 teaspoon freshly ground black pepper

Place all the ingredients in a blender and blend for 2 to 3 minutes until emulsified. Store in a tightly closed jar in the refrigerator.

Flaxseed Oil Salad Dressing

4 servings

4 tablespoons organic flaxseed oil
1½ tablespoons fresh lemon juice
1 garlic clove, crushed
Pinch of salt substitute
Freshly ground black pepper

Whisk together all the ingredients in a small bowl until smooth and creamy. Cover and refrigerate any leftovers.

....

Thai Salad

2 servings

Salad
1 small head romaine lettuce, chopped
1 red bell pepper, seeded and cut into strips
1 carrot, shredded
1⅓ cups bean sprouts
1 small cucumber, halved and sliced
⅔ cup snow peas, trimmed and cut into ½-inch pieces
¼ cup slivered red onions
⅓ cup chopped fresh cilantro
⅓ cup chopped fresh mint

Dressing
2 tablespoons fresh lime juice
1 tablespoon coconut oil
1 tablespoon Asian sesame oil
2 teaspoons xylitol or natural stevia-based sweetener, or to taste
1 teaspoon low-sodium soy sauce
1 garlic clove, minced
½ teaspoon cayenne pepper

Toss the salad ingredients together in a large salad bowl. In a small bowl, whisk together the dressing ingredients until the xylitol has dissolved. Gently toss the salad with the dressing and serve.

....

Greek Salad

2 servings

Salad

½ red bell pepper, seeded and cut into 1-inch pieces
¼ green bell pepper, seeded and cut into 1-inch pieces
½ cup cherry tomatoes, halved
½ cucumber, peeled and thickly sliced
½ red onion, thinly sliced
½ cup crumbled feta cheese
¼ cup pitted kalamata olives
1½ teaspoons capers, rinsed

Dressing

2 tablespoons red wine vinegar
1 small garlic clove, minced
1½ teaspoons minced fresh dill
¼ teaspoon dried oregano
¼ teaspoon salt substitute
¼ teaspoon freshly ground black pepper
1 tablespoon extra-virgin olive oil

In a large bowl, toss together the bell peppers, tomatoes, cucumber, onion, feta, olives, and capers. In a small bowl, whisk the vinegar, garlic, dill, oregano, salt substitute, and black pepper. While whisking, slowly drizzle in the oil to make a thick dressing. Pour the dressing over the salad, toss, and serve immediately.

....

Asparagus Salad

2 servings

Salad
½ pound fresh asparagus, trimmed
2 cups mixed salad greens

Dressing
3 tablespoons balsamic vinegar
1 tablespoon fresh orange juice
1 tablespoon sesame seed, toasted
1 teaspoon minced fresh ginger

Prepare an ice bath. Fill a skillet with enough water to cover the asparagus. Bring the water to a boil, add the asparagus, and cover the skillet. Boil for 3 to 5 minutes, depending on the thickness of the asparagus, or until the asparagus is crisp-tender. Using tongs, transfer the asparagus to a bowl of ice water. When cool, drain the water and pat the asparagus dry. Place the salad greens on a serving platter; top with the asparagus. In a small bowl, whisk together the vinegar, orange juice, sesame seed, and ginger. Drizzle over the salad.

....

Tomato Salad

2 servings

Salad
3 tomatoes, quartered
½ green bell pepper, seeded and thinly sliced
½ onion, thinly sliced and separated into rings
1 large cucumber, peeled and sliced

Dressing
¼ cup balsamic vinegar
½ teaspoon celery seed
½ teaspoon Dijon mustard
¼ teaspoon salt substitute
⅛ teaspoon freshly ground black pepper

In a large bowl, combine the tomatoes, bell pepper, and onion. In a small saucepan, combine the vinegar, celery seed, mustard, salt substitute, and black pepper; bring to a boil. Boil for 1 minute, then pour over the vegetables. Let stand until the mixture comes to room temperature. Stir in the cucumber. Cover and refrigerate for 2 hours before serving.

....

Jicama-Orange Salad

2 servings

Salad
1 small jicama, peeled and cut into ¼-inch-thick sticks
1 orange, peeled, sectioned, and cut into chunks
1 cucumber, seeded and thinly sliced
¼ cup chopped green onions (scallions)
¼ cup chopped fresh cilantro
1 tablespoon chopped fresh mint

Dressing
¼ cup fresh orange juice
¼ cup fresh lemon or lime juice
¼ teaspoon salt substitute
¼ teaspoon freshly ground black pepper
¼ teaspoon chili powder

Combine the jicama, orange pieces, cucumber, green onions, cilantro, and mint in a medium bowl. In a separate bowl, whisk together the orange juice, lemon juice, salt substitute, pepper, and chili powder. Toss the dressing with the jicama mixture. Cover and chill for 20 minutes before serving.

....

Cucumber-Fennel Salad

2 servings

Salad
1 large cucumber, sliced
½ sweet onion, thinly sliced
1 small fennel bulb, thinly sliced

Dressing
2 tablespoons fresh lemon juice
2 tablespoons extra-virgin olive oil
1 teaspoon chopped fresh dill
¼ teaspoon grated lemon zest
⅛ teaspoon freshly ground black pepper
⅛ teaspoon salt substitute

In a large bowl, combine the cucumber, onion, and fennel. In a jar with a tight-fitting lid, combine the lemon juice, oil, dill, lemon zest, pepper, and salt substitute; shake well. Pour the dressing over the cucumber mixture and toss to coat. Refrigerate until chilled.

Orange and Fennel Salad

2 servings

1 orange
1 small fennel bulb
1 small head romaine lettuce, cut up
¼ cup chopped fresh flat-leaf parsley
1 tablespoon Synergetic Salad Dressing (page 173)

Remove the peel and white pith from the orange. Slice the orange and fennel, then toss with the greens and dressing in a large bowl.

Simple Green Salad with Bell Peppers, Carrots, and Radishes

2 servings

4 cups mixed salad greens
1 green bell pepper, seeded and chopped
½ cup chopped carrots
½ cup chopped radishes
2 tablespoons Synergetic Salad Dressing (page 173)

Toss the salad greens, bell pepper, carrots, and radishes in a bowl. Add the dressing and toss well.

....

Black Bean and Corn Salad

2 servings

Salad
1 (15-ounce) can black beans, rinsed and drained
1 cup frozen corn, thawed
6 cherry tomatoes, quartered
½ cup minced green onions (scallions)
1 garlic clove, minced
½ cup seeded and diced red bell pepper
½ cup chopped fresh cilantro
2 cups mixed salad greens

Dressing
1 tablespoon extra-virgin olive oil
2 tablespoons fresh lemon juice
¼ cup chopped fresh cilantro
Salt substitute and freshly ground black pepper

Toss the salad ingredients in a large bowl. In a small bowl, whisk the oil, lemon juice, cilantro, salt substitute, and black pepper. Toss the salad with the dressing until well combined.

....

Mediterranean Salad

2 servings

1 tomato, chopped
1 cup chopped peeled cucumber
½ cup finely minced green onions (scallions)
1 garlic clove, finely minced
1 cup canned chickpeas, rinsed and drained
1 tablespoon fresh lemon juice
1 tablespoon chopped fresh flat-leaf parsley
1 teaspoon dried Italian seasoning
1 tablespoon extra-virgin olive oil

Mix all ingredients together in a large bowl and chill for at least 15 minutes.

....

Mediterranean Mint Salad

2 servings

Salad
3 tablespoons chopped fresh mint
2 small cucumbers, diced
4 plum tomatoes, diced
1 small red onion, minced
2 garlic cloves, minced
¼ cup pitted and sliced kalamata olives
½ cup crumbled feta cheese

Dressing
2 tablespoons extra-virgin olive oil
¼ cup fresh lemon juice
⅛ teaspoon salt substitute
⅛ teaspoon freshly ground black pepper

Toss the mint, cucumbers, tomatoes, onion, garlic, olives, and feta together in a large bowl. In a separate bowl, whisk the oil, lemon juice, salt substitute, and pepper. Combine the dressing with the salad and chill at least 3 hours.

....

Lima Bean–Tomato Salad

2 servings

Salad
2½ cups cooked lima beans, fresh or frozen
2 tablespoons minced onions
2 large plum tomatoes, seeded and chopped

Dressing
¼ cup apple cider vinegar
2 tablespoons coconut oil
1 garlic clove, minced
1 teaspoon Dijon mustard
½ teaspoon dried crumbled sage
¼ teaspoon freshly ground black pepper

Combine the lima beans, onions, and tomatoes in a large bowl. In a small bowl, whisk together the vinegar, oil, garlic, mustard, sage, and pepper. Toss the salad with the dressing and let sit for 1 hour before serving.

....

Chicken-Spinach Salad

2 servings

2 tomatoes, cut into bite-size pieces
3 cups fresh spinach leaves
8 ounces grilled or baked boneless, skinless chicken breast, cut into 1-inch cubes
½ cup coarsely chopped walnuts
1 tablespoon extra-virgin olive oil
1 tablespoon balsamic vinegar
⅛ teaspoon salt substitute

In a large bowl, toss the tomatoes with the spinach. Add the chicken, walnuts, oil, vinegar, and salt substitute and toss well.

....

Turkey Waldorf Salad

2 servings

8 ounces cooked turkey breast, cut into 1-inch cubes
1 apple, cored and chopped
1 cup sliced celery (about 2 small stalks)
1 cup halved red seedless grapes
½ cup coarsely chopped walnuts
⅓ cup reduced-fat mayonnaise
¼ teaspoon salt substitute
¼ teaspoon freshly ground black pepper
4 cups mixed salad greens
2 tablespoons chopped fresh flat-leaf parsley

In a large bowl, toss the turkey, apple, celery, grapes, walnuts, and mayonnaise. Season with the salt substitute and pepper. Serve on a bed of greens. Sprinkle with the parsley.

....

Soups and Stews

Soups and stews are hearty, filling, and they travel well, so you can pack them to go.

You can use nonfat plain yogurt for flavor or thickening, but avoid other dairy products, other than nonfat.

Red Bean and Tomato Soup

2 servings

½ cup chopped onions
1 garlic clove, minced
1 celery stalk, chopped
1 tablespoon extra-virgin olive oil
1 cup red kidney beans, rinsed and drained
1 (10.75-ounce) can low-sodium tomato soup
2 tablespoons dried Italian seasoning

Salt substitute and freshly ground black pepper
2 Ryvita or Wasa whole grain rye crackers

In a medium saucepan, sauté the onions, garlic, and celery in the oil over medium-low heat until the vegetables are soft, about 5 minutes. Put the beans, tomato soup, and Italian seasoning in a blender and puree until smooth. Add the bean mixture and 1 cup water to the vegetables. Cook, stirring occasionally, for 15 minutes. Season with salt substitute and pepper. Serve 1 cracker with each bowlful.

....

Italian White Bean Soup

2 servings

½ onion, thinly sliced
1 tablespoon extra-virgin olive oil
4 garlic cloves, sliced
2 cups chicken or vegetable broth
2 cups finely chopped collard greens or kale leaves
1 cup diced tomatoes, fresh or canned
2 teaspoons dried Italian seasoning
1 (15-ounce) can navy or small white beans, rinsed and drained
Salt substitute and freshly ground black pepper, to taste

Sauté the onion in the olive oil in a medium saucepan over medium-low heat for 5 minutes, stirring frequently. Add the garlic and continue to sauté for another minute. Add the broth, greens, tomatoes, and Italian seasoning. Simmer for 15 minutes over medium heat. Stir in the beans and cook for another 5 minutes. Season with salt substitute and pepper.

....

Turkish Red Lentil Soup

2 servings

1 cup red lentils, picked over and rinsed
2 cups vegetable broth
1 small russet potato, peeled and diced
¼ cup finely chopped onions
2 teaspoons ground cumin
1 teaspoon paprika
½ teaspoon dried mint
½ teaspoon dried thyme or oregano
Salt substitute, to taste
¼ teaspoon freshly ground black pepper

In a medium saucepan, combine the lentils, broth, potato, onions, cumin, paprika, mint, thyme, salt substitute, and pepper. Bring the soup to a boil, then reduce to a simmer. Loosely place a lid on the pan and cook for 40 to 45 minutes, until the lentils are tender, stirring occasionally. Then place all but 1 cup of the soup into a blender or food processor and blend briefly. Return the blended soup to the saucepan. Heat through.

....

Turkey Meatballs and Tomato Soup

2 servings

1 cup chicken broth
1 (14.5-ounce) can diced tomatoes
1 tablespoon tomato paste
½ cup quick-cooking brown rice
1 garlic clove, minced
¼ teaspoon caraway seed (optional)
8 ounces extra-lean ground turkey breast
⅛ teaspoon salt substitute
⅛ teaspoon freshly ground black pepper
1 tablespoon chopped fresh basil leaves

Put the broth, tomatoes, and tomato paste into a large heavy saucepan and bring to a boil. Add the rice and cook, stirring briskly, for 5 minutes. Reduce the heat to a simmer. Meanwhile, in a medium bowl, combine the garlic, caraway seed, turkey, salt substitute, and pepper. Mix well. Divide and shape the mixture into 16 balls. Using a slotted spoon, carefully lower the meatballs into the tomato soup. Simmer for 8 to 10 minutes, until the turkey balls and rice are cooked. Garnish each serving with some basil.

....

Creamy Chickpea and Rosemary Soup

2 servings

1 tablespoon extra-virgin olive oil
2 garlic cloves, minced
1½ teaspoons minced fresh rosemary leaves
½ teaspoon crushed red pepper flakes
1 (15-ounce) can chickpeas, rinsed and drained
2 cups chicken or vegetable broth
1 tablespoon fresh lemon juice
Salt substitute, to taste

In a large saucepan, heat the oil over medium heat. Add the garlic, rosemary, and red pepper flakes. Cook, stirring constantly, until the garlic starts to brown, about 1 minute. Add the chickpeas and cook for 2 minutes, stirring constantly. Add the broth and bring to a boil. Reduce the heat and simmer for 20 minutes. Let the soup cool slightly, then transfer it to a blender. Puree until smooth. Return to the saucepan and reheat. Stir in the lemon juice and salt substitute.

....

Spicy Black Bean Soup

2 servings

1 tablespoon extra-virgin olive oil
1 onion, chopped
2 garlic cloves, minced
1 teaspoon dried thyme
1 (15-ounce) can black beans, rinsed and drained
2 cups chicken or vegetable broth
1 cup diced tomatoes, fresh or canned
1 teaspoon ground cumin
½ teaspoon Tabasco sauce

In a large saucepan, heat the oil over medium heat. Add the onion and cook until soft and translucent. Add the garlic and thyme and cook for 2 minutes more. Add the beans, broth, tomatoes, cumin, and Tabasco and bring to a boil. Reduce the heat to medium-low, cover, and simmer for 20 to 30 minutes; stirring occasionally. Remove 3 cups of the soup from the pot and puree it in a blender until smooth. Return the pureed soup to the saucepan and reheat until hot.

....

Bean and Kale Soup

2 servings

1 tablespoon extra-virgin olive oil
2 garlic cloves, minced
½ yellow onion, chopped
2 cups chopped kale leaves, rinsed but not dried
2 cups chicken or vegetable broth
1 cup cannellini or other white beans, rinsed and drained
1 cup diced tomatoes, fresh or canned
1 teaspoon dried Italian seasoning
⅛ teaspoon salt substitute
⅛ teaspoon freshly ground black pepper
½ cup chopped fresh flat-leaf parsley

In a large saucepan, heat the oil. Add the garlic and onion; sauté until soft. Add the kale to the saucepan and cook until wilted. Stir in the broth, beans, tomatoes, Italian seasoning, salt substitute, and pepper. Cook until heated through. Garnish with the parsley.

....

Tuscan White Bean Soup

2 servings

½ shallot, finely diced
½ garlic clove, minced
1 tablespoon extra-virgin olive oil
1½ to 2 cups chicken or vegetable broth
1 cup diced tomatoes, fresh or canned
1 cup white beans, such as cannellini, rinsed and drained

½ teaspoon dried rosemary
Salt substitute and freshly ground black pepper, to taste
Crushed red pepper flakes, to taste

In a large saucepan, sauté the shallot and garlic in the oil. Add the broth, tomatoes, beans, and rosemary. Season with salt substitute, black pepper, and red pepper flakes. Bring to a boil, reduce the heat, and simmer for 2 minutes. If the soup seems too thick, add a bit more broth.

....

Vegetable Soup

2 servings

1 tablespoon extra-virgin olive oil
2 carrots, cut into 1-inch slices
2 celery stalks, thinly sliced
1 large onion, chopped
1 garlic clove, minced
1 (8-ounce) can tomato sauce
½ head cauliflower, cut into bite-size pieces
1 zucchini, cut into 1-inch chunks
1 (5-ounce) package fresh spinach leaves, rinsed
½ cup chopped fresh flat-leaf parsley
4 cups chicken or vegetable broth
½ teaspoon freshly ground black pepper
1 teaspoon salt substitute

In a large saucepan, heat the oil over medium heat. Add the carrots, celery, onion, and garlic. Sauté, stirring occasionally, until soft, about 5 minutes. Stir in the tomato sauce. Add the cauliflower, zucchini, spinach, parsley, broth, pepper, and salt substitute. Bring to a boil, stirring occasionally. Reduce the heat to low; cover and simmer, stirring occasionally, for 15 to 20 minutes, or until the vegetables are tender. Taste and add more salt substitute and pepper if needed. Note: the serving size for this soup is large, but the calorie content is quite low.

....

Black Bean Chili

2 servings

½ onion, chopped
2 garlic cloves, minced
1 green bell pepper, seeded and diced
1 tablespoon extra-virgin olive oil
1 cup chicken or vegetable broth
1 (15-ounce) can black beans, rinsed and drained
1 cup frozen corn kernels
½ cup tomato sauce
2 tablespoons chili powder
1 tablespoon ground cumin
1 tablespoon dried Italian seasoning
Salt substitute and freshly ground black pepper, to taste
¼ cup chopped fresh cilantro
2 whole wheat tortillas, heated

Combine the onion, garlic, bell pepper, and oil in a medium saucepan over medium-low heat, cook until the vegetables are tender, stirring frequently, for 5 minutes. Add the broth, beans, corn, tomato sauce, chili powder, cumin, Italian seasoning, salt substitute, and pepper and simmer for 15 minutes. Divide between 2 bowls and garnish with the cilantro. Serve with the whole wheat tortillas.

....

White Chicken Chili

2 servings

1 tablespoon olive oil
8 ounces boneless, skinless chicken breast, cubed
1 (14.5-ounce) can chicken broth
1 small onion, chopped
1 garlic clove, minced
½ (4-ounce) can chopped green chiles
1 (15-ounce) can white beans, rinsed and drained
½ teaspoon ground cumin
½ teaspoon dried oregano

¼ teaspoon freshly ground black pepper
¼ teaspoon salt substitute
⅛ teaspoon cayenne pepper
2 to 3 green onions (scallions), thinly sliced, for garnish

Heat the oil in a nonstick skillet over medium heat. Add the chicken and sauté until lightly browned; remove from the heat and set aside. Pour half the chicken broth into a large saucepan and add the onion and garlic. Bring to a simmer and cook until the onion softens. Add the chiles, stir, then add the remaining broth and the beans. Stir in the cumin, oregano, black pepper, salt substitute, and cayenne. Bring to a boil, reduce the heat to a simmer, and add the chicken. Cover and simmer for 30 to 45 minutes. Garnish with the green onions.

....

Turkey Tacos

4 servings

1 tablespoon extra-virgin olive oil
1 cup diced onions
1 to 2 garlic cloves, minced
3 cups diced or shredded cooked turkey or chicken
1 (1.25-ounce) package taco seasoning mix
2 (14.5-ounce) cans diced tomatoes with juice
1 (15-ounce) can black beans or kidney beans, rinsed and drained
1 (8.75-ounce) can whole kernel corn, rinsed and drained
1 (4-ounce) can diced green chiles, drained
1½ teaspoons cornstarch
1 cup chicken broth
4 whole wheat tortillas

Heat the oil in a large saucepan over medium heat. Add the onions and garlic and sauté until tender. Add the turkey, taco seasoning, tomatoes, beans, corn, and chiles. Whisk the cornstarch into the broth until dissolved and then stir into the chili. Bring to a boil; reduce the heat and simmer for 15 minutes, stirring occasionally. Serve with the tortillas.

....

Black Bean–Chicken Chili

4 servings

2 boneless, skinless chicken breast halves, cut into 1-inch pieces
1 cup chopped onions
1 cup chopped green bell peppers
2 garlic cloves, minced
2 tablespoons chicken broth
2 (14.5-ounce) cans stewed tomatoes
1 (15-ounce) can black beans, rinsed and drained
1 teaspoon salt substitute
½ teaspoon hot sauce, or to taste
2 cups medium tomato salsa
2 tablespoons chili powder
1 teaspoon ground cumin
Shredded low-fat cheddar cheese, for garnish (optional)
Nonfat plain yogurt, for garnish (optional)

Simmer the chicken, onions, bell peppers, and garlic in the broth in a covered large saucepan until the chicken is cooked through, 10 to 15 minutes. Add the tomatoes, beans, salt substitute, hot sauce, salsa, chili powder, and cumin; mix well and simmer for 30 to 45 minutes. Garnish with the cheese or yogurt, if desired.

....

Kidney Bean, Barley, and Sweet Potato Stew

2 servings

1 cup vegetable broth, plus more as needed
2 tablespoons pearl barley
1 cup canned kidney beans, rinsed and drained
1 small onion, diced
1 small sweet potato, peeled and diced
1 small celery stalk, diced
⅛ teaspoon freshly ground black pepper
¼ teaspoon salt substitute
⅛ teaspoon dried thyme, crushed
¼ teaspoon dried sage

In a medium saucepan, bring the broth to a boil. Stir in the barley, reduce the heat, and cover. Simmer for 30 minutes, stirring occasionally. Add the beans, onion, sweet potato, celery, pepper, salt substitute, thyme, and sage and simmer, covered, for 20 minutes, or until the vegetables are tender. Stir occasionally, and add more broth if the stew dries out.

....

Lebanese Chicken Stew

2 servings

3 teaspoons extra-virgin olive oil
8 ounces boneless, skinless chicken breast, cubed
1 small leek, white part only, thinly sliced
1 garlic clove, crushed
¼ teaspoon grated fresh ginger
1 small red onion, quartered
¼ teaspoon saffron threads
¼ teaspoon ground cinnamon
¼ teaspoon ground ginger
¾ cup chicken broth
1 small tomato, seeded and diced
1 dried date, seeded and minced, or 10 raisins, minced
1 tablespoon fresh lemon juice
Salt substitute and freshly ground black pepper, to taste

Heat 2 teaspoons of the oil in a large saucepan. Add the chicken and sauté until browned. Transfer to a plate. Heat the remaining 1 teaspoon oil and then add the leek, garlic, fresh ginger, and onion. Sauté until soft, 5 to 8 minutes. Add the saffron, cinnamon, ground ginger, and broth. Cover the pot and simmer for 20 minutes. Return the chicken to the pot along with the tomato and date and simmer for 30 to 40 minutes, or until the chicken is tender. Add the lemon juice. Season with salt substitute and pepper.

....

Midafternoon Snacks

For me, a midafternoon snack is a low-calorie fresh juice, especially during the summer.

Dinner

Here are some simple, important guidelines when constructing your main meal of the day:

- Create volume. To help you feel full, fill up on nonstarchy vegetables. These are considered "free" since they are high in fiber and low in calories. Avoid big portions of root vegetables such as white potatoes and parsnips.

- Go for low-glycemic-index foods. Choose fruits and vegetables that will not cause your blood sugar level to spike.

- Aim for balance. When creating a balanced meal, include choices from three or four food groups.

- Lower the fat. Avoid frying or deep-frying foods and using lots of fat. When cooking, try baking, broiling, grilling, poaching, roasting, sautéing with little oil, steaming, or stir-frying.

- Use nonstick cookware. Nonstick pans allow you to reduce calories by cooking food with little or no fat.

- Trim off any fat on meat and use skinless chicken or turkey breasts.

Dinner menus can feature some of the same recipes given for lunch. At every dinner, enjoy a fresh salad and a low-calorie vegetable side dish, especially if you're trying to lose weight.

Asian Salmon

2 servings

2 (4-ounce) salmon fillets
2 teaspoons low-sodium soy sauce
1 tablespoon Dijon mustard
½ cup sliced onions
1 garlic clove, minced
1½ teaspoons minced fresh ginger
2 cups stemmed and sliced fresh shiitake mushrooms

Preheat the oven to 375°F. Put the salmon into a baking dish. In a small bowl, whisk the soy sauce and mustard. Spread the mixture on the salmon. In a medium nonstick skillet, sauté the onions, garlic, ginger, and mushrooms until browned, about 5 minutes. Bake the salmon, depending on how thick it is (about 7 minutes if less than 1 inch thick). When cooked, place on a bed of sautéed mushrooms.

....

Tuna Salad Wrap

2 servings

1 (5-ounce) can white tuna, packed in water, drained
¼ cup minced onions
1 celery stalk, chopped
2 tablespoons Dijon mustard
1 tablespoon extra-virgin olive oil
1 tablespoon chopped fresh flat-leaf parsley
1 teaspoon fresh lemon juice
½ teaspoon salt substitute
½ teaspoon freshly ground black pepper
2 whole wheat tortillas or 2 slices whole grain bread

Mix the tuna, onions, celery, mustard, oil, parsley, lemon juice, salt substitute, and pepper in a small bowl. Spoon onto the tortillas and roll up. Or make 2 open-faced sandwiches with whole grain bread.

....

Thai-Style Tilapia

2 servings

¼ cup light coconut milk
3 whole almonds
½ small white onion, chopped
½ teaspoon ground ginger
⅛ teaspoon ground turmeric
½ teaspoon chopped fresh lemongrass or grated lemon zest
⅛ teaspoon salt substitute, plus more for seasoning
2 (4-ounce) tilapia, red snapper, or flounder fillets
⅛ teaspoon freshly ground black pepper
¼ teaspoon crushed red pepper flakes

In a food processor or blender, combine the coconut milk, almonds, onion, ginger, turmeric, lemongrass, and salt substitute. Process until smooth. Heat a large nonstick skillet over medium-high heat. Season the fish fillets with salt substitute and black pepper on both sides, then place them skin side up in the skillet. Pour the pureed sauce over the fish. Using a spatula, coat the fish evenly with the sauce. Sprinkle with red pepper flakes. Reduce the heat to medium, cover, and simmer for about 15 minutes, until the puree is thickened and the fish flakes easily with a fork.

....

Halibut with Vegetables

2 servings

Cooking oil spray
1 tablespoon extra-virgin olive oil
1 small zucchini, sliced
½ small onion, sliced
½ cup sliced mushrooms
2 lemon slices
⅛ teaspoon freshly ground black pepper
Large pinch of garlic powder
2 (6-ounce) halibut, red snapper, or cod fillets

Preheat the oven to 375°F. Spray a baking dish large enough to hold the fish in a single layer with cooking oil spray. Heat the oil in a skillet. Add the zucchini, onion, mushrooms, and lemon slices and sauté until tender, about 5 minutes. Remove the lemon slices and set aside. Stir the pepper and garlic powder into the vegetables. Place the fish in the baking dish and top with the vegetables and lemon slices. Bake for 15 to 20 minutes.

....

Grilled Salmon with Horseradish and Soy Sauce

2 servings

1 tablespoon low-sodium soy sauce
2 teaspoons prepared horseradish
2 (6-ounce) salmon fillets
Cooking oil spray

In a small bowl, whisk the soy sauce and horseradish. Spoon over the salmon, cover, and refrigerate for 1 to 2 hours. Heat a grill pan to medium. Spray the grill pan with the cooking oil spray. Grill the fish for 3 to 4 minutes on each side.

....

Curried Tofu or Chicken with Brown Rice

2 servings

½ cup quick-cooking brown rice
1½ ounces firm tofu, or 1 boneless, skinless chicken breast
1 tablespoon extra-virgin olive oil
½ cup chopped onions
1 garlic clove, minced
½ teaspoon ground ginger
2 teaspoons curry powder
1 cup chicken or vegetable broth
1 bell pepper, seeded and chopped
½ cup coconut milk, stirred
Salt substitute and freshly ground black pepper, to taste

Follow the instructions on the package of quick brown rice. While the water for the rice is coming to a boil, cut the tofu into small cubes. Heat the oil in a medium skillet. Add the onions and sauté until soft, about 5 minutes. Add the garlic and ginger and continue to sauté for another minute. Remove the skillet from the heat and stir in the curry powder. Return the skillet to the heat and add the broth, tofu, bell pepper, and coconut milk. Simmer until the tofu is done, about 10 minutes. Season with salt substitute and pepper, and serve the curry with a scoop of rice.

....

Polenta Puttanesca with Tofu

2 servings

Sauce
1 tablespoon extra-virgin olive oil
1 onion, diced
1 garlic clove, crushed or minced
1 green bell pepper, seeded and diced
1½ cups tomato sauce
7½ ounces firm tofu, cut into small cubes
1 tablespoon dried Italian seasoning
1 bay leaf
1 teaspoon crushed red pepper flakes
2 tablespoons capers, rinsed and drained
4 to 6 pitted kalamata olives, coarsely chopped
1 tablespoon finely chopped fresh flat-leaf parsley
¼ teaspoon salt substitute
½ teaspoon ground black pepper

Polenta
1 teaspoon salt substitute
1 cup instant polenta

Sauce: In a large saucepan, heat the olive oil over medium heat. Add the onion and garlic and sauté until soft, 3 to 4 minutes. Add the bell pepper and sauté for 3 to 4 minutes more. Add 1 cup water and bring to a boil. Cover the pot and simmer for 15 minutes. Add the tomato sauce, tofu, Italian seasoning, bay leaf, red pepper flakes, capers, olives, parsley, salt substitute, and black pepper and simmer for 15 minutes, stirring occasionally. Remove and discard the bay leaf.

Polenta: Bring 3 cups water to a boil in a medium saucepan. Add the salt substitute and reduce the heat until the water is simmering. Slowly pour in the polenta, simultaneously stirring with a wooden spoon to avoid lumps. Cook, stirring continuously, for 5 minutes, or until the polenta is solid but still soft. Pour into large bowls or plates. Let cool about 10 minutes, or until firm, before pouring on the sauce.

Spicy Black Bean and Lentil Burgers

4 servings

1 (15-ounce) can black beans, rinsed and drained
1 (15-ounce) can lentils, rinsed and drained
½ small onion, finely chopped
1 to 2 jalapeño peppers, seeded and minced
2 teaspoons chili powder
2 teaspoons salt substitute
1 teaspoon freshly ground black pepper
2 large eggs, beaten
½ cup dry bread crumbs
Cooking oil spray

Mash the beans and lentils well in a large bowl. Stir in the onion, jalapeños, chili powder, salt substitute, black pepper, eggs, and bread crumbs. Shape the mixture into 8 patties. Spray a large skillet with the cooking spray and heat over medium-high heat. Place the patties in the skillet and cook until firm and browned, about 5 minutes per side.

Garlic-Lime Grilled Chicken with Mango Salsa

2 servings

2 boneless, skinless chicken breast halves
1 tablespoon extra-virgin olive oil
Juice of 1 large lime
2 garlic cloves, minced

Salsa
2 ripe mangoes, peeled, pitted, and chopped
2 ripe plum tomatoes, chopped
½ red or yellow bell pepper, seeded and chopped
½ serrano chile, seeded and minced (or to taste)
1 green onion (scallion), thinly sliced
⅛ cup chopped fresh cilantro
Juice of ½ lime
Salt substitute and freshly ground black pepper, to taste

2 cups cooked instant brown rice

Put the chicken, oil, lime juice, and garlic into a resealable bag. Close the bag and shake to distribute the marinade. Refrigerate for at least 2 hours or overnight. For the salsa, mix all the ingredients together in a bowl. Preheat a grill or grill pan. Discard the marinade. Grill the chicken breast, until done, about 5 minutes per side. Divide the rice and chicken between two plates and top with the salsa.

....

Grilled Chipotle-Lime Chicken Breasts

2 servings

¼ cup canned chipotles in adobo, minced
½ teaspoon adobo sauce from canned chipotles
2 tablespoons fresh lime juice
½ garlic clove, minced
1 tablespoon extra-virgin olive oil
⅛ teaspoon salt substitute
⅛ teaspoon freshly ground black pepper
2 boneless, skinless chicken breast halves

Whisk the chipotles, adobo sauce, lime juice, garlic, oil, salt substitute, and black pepper in a small bowl. Reserve half of the marinade. Pour the remaining marinade and the chicken into a resealable bag. Marinate for 15 minutes. Preheat a grill or grill pan to medium-high. Remove the chicken from the marinade (discard the marinade) and place on the grill. Baste the chicken with the remaining marinade and grill the chicken on both sides until done, 4 to 5 minutes per side. Serve the chicken with any remaining marinade.

....

Lemon Turkey Scaloppini

2 servings

1 tablespoon extra-virgin olive oil
1 tablespoon all-purpose flour
⅛ teaspoon salt substitute
⅛ teaspoon freshly ground black pepper
2 (8-ounce) turkey breast cutlets, pounded ¼ inch thick
1 tablespoon fresh lemon juice
1 tablespoon minced fresh flat-leaf parsley

Heat the oil in a large nonstick skillet. Combine the flour, salt substitute, and pepper on a plate. Coat the turkey cutlets with the seasoned flour, shaking off any excess. Place the cutlets in the skillet and cook for 1 to 2 minutes per side, until browned. Transfer to a plate lined with paper towels to drain. Reduce the heat to medium. Add the lemon juice and parsley to the skillet, stirring with a wooden spoon to loosen the browned bits in the pan. Return the cutlets to the skillet and cook for 1 to 2 minutes, until heated through, basting often with the lemon-parsley sauce.

....

Turkey à l'Orange

2 servings

1 large orange, cut in half crosswise
¼ cup chicken broth
¾ teaspoon cornstarch
1 tablespoon extra-virgin olive oil
2 (4-ounce) turkey breast cutlets, pounded ½ inch thick
Salt substitute and freshly ground black pepper, to taste

Squeeze 2 tablespoons of juice from half of the orange. Peel and cut the remaining half into ¼-inch-thick slices and set aside. In a small bowl, whisk the orange juice, broth, and cornstarch to dissolve. In a large nonstick skillet, heat the oil. Season the turkey cutlets with salt substitute and pepper. Place the cutlets into the skillet and cook for 5 to 8 minutes per side. Transfer the cutlets to a platter to keep warm. Add the orange slices to the skillet and cook for 2 minutes. Transfer the orange slices to the platter with the cutlets. Stir the juice-cornstarch mix into the skillet and bring to a boil. Return the cutlets and orange slices to the skillet to warm through.

Chicken or Turkey Burgers

2 servings

8 ounces extra-lean ground chicken or ground turkey breast
2 tablespoons ketchup
2 tablespoons seasoned dry bread crumbs
1 tablespoon grated onion
1 large egg white
1 garlic clove, minced
¼ teaspoon salt substitute
¼ teaspoon freshly ground black pepper
2 (¼-inch) slices red or yellow onion
Cooking oil spray

Preheat a grill or grill pan. In a large bowl, combine the ground chicken, ketchup, bread crumbs, onion, egg white, garlic, salt substitute, and pepper. Mix well and shape into 2 patties about ½ inch thick. Coat the patties and onion slices with cooking oil spray. Grill the patties and onion over medium heat until cooked through, 6 to 7 minutes per side.

Evening Snack

Do you have to eat an evening snack? Not necessarily, but some of us do benefit from one. What changed my philosophy on this matter was seeing the effect of a nighttime feeding on my kids when they were babies. They seemed to sleep much better on a full stomach. I think the same is true for many adults. The key is to avoid eating high-glycemic foods, which will promote a blood sugar roller coaster.

For many years I tried not to eat anything after dinner, but I wasn't successful. Like others, I was able to stick to my diet during the day, but when I ate dinner, it triggered a hormonal reaction that felt as though the more I ate, the hungrier I became. For me, PGX was a godsend. I regularly have a nighttime snack of 5 grams of PGX in some instant oatmeal or mixed with non-fat Greek yogurt and ground flaxseed or berries and some xylitol to sweeten it. This evening snack helps me achieve my dietary goals and sleep soundly through the night.

I also drink a cup of relaxing caffeine-free herbal tea at night. Choose from a variety of teas such as rooibos, peppermint, chamomile, ginger, and decaffeinated English breakfast.

Vegetable Side Dishes

When raw, vegetables are easy to snack on or make salads with, but cooking them brings out their flavors. Use these recipes to accompany other dishes or make several for a vegetarian meal.

Dr. Murray's Favorite Greens

2 servings

1 tablespoon extra-virgin olive oil
1 teaspoon balsamic vinegar
1 large bunch kale, collards, or other greens,
    stemmed, washed, and coarsely chopped
½ cup diced green onions (scallions)
1 garlic clove, thinly sliced
½ cup coarsely chopped walnuts or almonds
¼ teaspoon salt substitute
½ teaspoon freshly ground black pepper
Lemon wedges

Heat the oil and vinegar in a large skillet. Add the kale, green onions, garlic, and walnuts and sauté until soft, about 5 minutes. Season with salt substitute and pepper. Serve with the lemon wedges.

....

Minted Carrots with Pumpkin Seeds

2 servings

3 carrots, cut into ½-inch rounds
1 tablespoon chopped fresh flat-leaf parsley
1 tablespoon chopped fresh mint
2 tablespoons coarsely chopped pumpkin seeds
1 tablespoon fresh lemon juice
1 tablespoon extra-virgin olive oil
Salt substitute and freshly ground black pepper, to taste

Steam the carrots until still slightly crunchy. Toss in a medium bowl with the parsley, mint, pumpkin seeds, lemon juice, and oil and season with salt substitute and pepper.

....

Oven-Roasted Vegetables

2 servings

1 zucchini, cut into 1-inch pieces
1 summer squash, cut into 1-inch pieces
1 red bell pepper, seeded and cut into 1-inch pieces
1 yellow bell pepper, seeded and cut into 1-inch pieces
1 pound fresh asparagus, trimmed and cut into 1-inch pieces
1 red onion, sliced
3 tablespoons extra-virgin olive oil
1 teaspoon salt substitute
¼ teaspoon freshly ground black pepper

Preheat the oven to 425°F. Arrange the vegetables in a single layer in a large baking dish. Add the oil, salt substitute, and black pepper and toss. Roast for 20 to 25 minutes, stirring occasionally, until the vegetables are crisp and browned.

....

Green Beans with Garlic and Lemon

2 servings

1 pound fresh green beans, trimmed
2 tablespoons extra-virgin olive oil
1 red onion, cut into thin wedges
2 garlic cloves, thinly sliced
3 tablespoons fresh lemon juice
1 teaspoon salt substitute
¼ teaspoon freshly ground black pepper

Put the green beans and 1 tablespoon water in a microwave-safe dish. Partially cover the dish and microwave the beans for 4 minutes on high. Heat the oil in a large skillet over medium heat. Add the onion and garlic and sauté until lightly browned. Add the green beans and 2 tablespoons of the lemon juice and cook until tender, stirring occasionally. Stir in the salt substitute and pepper. Sprinkle with the remaining 1 tablespoon lemon juice.

....

Cherry Tomato and Zucchini Sauté

2 servings

1 tablespoon extra-virgin olive oil
3 small zucchini, halved lengthwise and thinly sliced
2 cups cherry tomatoes, halved
2 green onions (scallions), sliced
2 teaspoons balsamic vinegar
¼ teaspoon salt substitute
⅛ teaspoon freshly ground black pepper
2 tablespoons chopped fresh basil, for garnish

Heat the oil in a large nonstick skillet over high heat. Add the zucchini and sauté, stirring, for 1 minute. Add the tomatoes, green onions, and vinegar. Cook, stirring, for 1 to 2 minutes, or until the zucchini is crisp-tender and the tomatoes are heated through. Season with salt substitute and pepper. Garnish with the basil and serve immediately.

....

Roasted Broccoli with Lemon and Garlic

2 servings

1 pound broccoli, cut into florets
2 tablespoons extra-virgin olive oil
2 tablespoons fresh lemon juice
¼ teaspoon salt substitute
⅛ teaspoon freshly ground black pepper
1 teaspoon minced garlic
½ teaspoon grated lemon zest

Preheat the oven to 425°F. In a large bowl, toss the broccoli with 1 tablespoon of the oil, 1 tablespoon of the lemon juice, the salt substitute, and pepper. Arrange the florets in a single layer in a baking dish and roast, turning once, for 15 minutes, until crisp-tender. Meanwhile, in a small saucepan, heat the remaining 1 tablespoon oil, the garlic, and lemon zest. Cook, stirring, for 1 minute. Let cool slightly and stir in the remaining 1 tablespoon lemon juice. Place the broccoli in a large bowl, pour the lemon dressing over it, and toss to coat.

....

Asparagus with Thyme

2 servings

1 garlic clove, halved
1½ pounds asparagus, trimmed
1 tablespoon extra-virgin olive oil
¼ teaspoon dried thyme
¼ teaspoon salt substitute
¼ teaspoon freshly ground black pepper

Preheat the oven to 400°F. Rub the cut sides of the garlic on the inside of a baking dish large enough to hold the asparagus in a single layer. Add the garlic and asparagus to the dish. Drizzle with the oil. Rotate the asparagus to coat with the oil. Sprinkle the asparagus with the thyme, salt substitute, and pepper. Toss gently and bake for 20 minutes, stirring once.

Sweet Treats

Focus on berries, mangoes, or other low-glycemic fresh fruits and some nonfat plain yogurt. If you want something a bit more satisfying, try one of these easy-to-make puddings.

Chocolate Chia Pudding

Serves 2

2 cups coconut milk
¼ cup chia seeds
2 tablespoons raw cacao powder
Dash of pure vanilla extract
1 teaspoon stevia

Combine the coconut milk and chia seeds in a blender and blend on low speed for 2 minutes. Add the cacao powder, vanilla extract, and stevia and blend on low speed for another 2 minutes. Pour into a bowl, cover, and refrigerate overnight before serving.

Raw Avocado Cacao Mousse

Serves 2

⅓ cup almond milk
1 avocado, pitted and peeled
½ cup raw cacao powder
2 teaspoons stevia

Place the almond milk and avocado in a blender and blend on medium speed until smooth. Then gradually add the cacao powder 1 tablespoon at a time. If needed, stop the blender to scrape down the sides with a spatula. Pour into a bowl, cover, and refrigerate for 6 to 8 hours.

....

A Four-Day Meal Plan

Day 1

Breakfast
- 1 cup organic egg whites and 1 whole egg with 3 tablespoons fresh herbs (dill, rosemary, thyme, basil, etc.) scrambled in 1 tablespoon avocado or extra-virgin olive oil
- 1 large tomato, sliced, drizzled with extra-virgin olive oil and balsamic vinegar

Midmorning Snack
- ¼ cup almonds
- 1 cup blueberries

Lunch
- Simple mixed green salad with healthy oil dressing
- Red Bean and Tomato Soup

Midafternoon Snack
- Go Green Drink

Dinner
- Asian Salmon
- Minted Carrots with Pumpkin Seeds
- Steamed broccoli
- ½ cup raspberries

Day 2

Breakfast
- Apple-Cinnamon Smoothie

Midmorning Snack
- Color Me Pink

Lunch
- Chicken-Spinach Salad

Midafternoon Snack
- 1 apple
- ¼ cup Brazil nuts

Dinner
- Turkey Tacos
- Jicama-Orange Salad
- ½ cup blueberries

Day 3

Breakfast
- Mediterranean Omelet

Midmorning Snack
- Fennel Citrus Mix

Lunch
- Italian White Bean Soup

Midafternoon Snack
- 8 ounces raw cut-up carrots, celery, and/or cucumbers

Dinner
- Thai-Style Tilapia
- Orange and Fennel Salad
- Chocolate Chia Pudding

Day 4

Breakfast
- Berry Smoothie

Midmorning Snack
- ¼ to ½ cup mixed nuts and seeds

Lunch
- Turkey Waldorf Salad

Midafternoon Snack
- Better Red Than Dead

Dinner
- Asparagus Salad
- Halibut with Vegetables
- Dr. Murray's Favorite Greens
- ½ cup blackberries

Food as Medicine

Many medical conditions respond well to nutritional interventions, because delivering improved nutrition to cells often addresses the underlying causes of the illness rather than simply covering up the symptoms.

The following dietary recommendations are not designed to be substitutes for proper medical treatment. In all cases involving a physical or medical complaint, ailment, or therapy, please consult a physician or health care provider with nutritional experience. For more information on natural approaches to more than a hundred different health conditions, please consult *The Encyclopedia of Natural Medicine*.

Acne

Acne is associated with a diet high in refined carbohydrates, dairy products, and the wrong types of fats. In Westernized societies, acne afflicts 79% to 95% of teenagers. In men and women older than 25 years, 40% to 54% still have some degree of facial acne. In contrast, acne is rare in populations who consume healthy traditional diets.

Despite the now-overwhelming scientific evidence linking diet and acne, many dermatologists still cling to the myth that diet has no impact on acne. They are wrong.

Acne is a sign of localized insulin resistance in the skin. In fact, in the early 1940s, some dermatologists began referring to acne as "skin diabetes." Although oral glucose tolerance tests in acne patients showed no differences from controls in blood glucose measurements, when researchers looked at the levels of glucose within the skin through repetitive biopsies, it revealed that the acne patients' skin glucose tolerance was significantly disturbed.

Anything that leads to a transient increase in skin sugar levels can worsen acne. This includes ingesting a high-sugar beverage or meal; the effects of stress (cortisol); a deficiency of nutrients necessary for proper utilization of insulin and glucose; and other factors that adversely affect blood sugar control (e.g., abdominal obesity).

Milk and other dairy products are a significant problem for many acne sufferers. In addition to detrimental fats, dairy products contain hormones that can increase sebum production, as well as promote an increase in insulin-like growth factor 1 (IGF-1), the major growth hormone of puberty. The acne-promoting effects of IGF-1 on the skin are related to dietary factors, especially too much refined sugar and dairy products. Acne sufferers are also sensitive to too much iodine, so I tell patients with acne to eliminate foods high in iodized salt from their diets—which means basically all processed foods, especially soups, crackers, tortillas, potato chips, etc.

Increasing the intake of foods high in zinc—nuts, whole grains, and legumes—and/or taking 30 to 45 mg of absorbable zinc picolinate daily has produced good results in double-blind studies.

More than 80% of the participants who took brewer's yeast in a double-blind study completely healed or considerably improved after five months of use, while the corresponding figure among those receiving a placebo was only 26%. The benefits of brewer's yeast may be due to the trace mineral chromium. High-chromium yeast is known to improve glucose tolerance and enhance insulin sensitivity and has been reported in an uncontrolled study to induce rapid improvement in patients with acne. The target dosage is 400 mcg of chromium per day.

Alzheimer's Disease

The Synergetic Diet offers the best approach to preventing Alzheimer's disease (AD). The closest diet to the Synergetic Diet that has been researched as a preventive approach to AD is the MIND (Mediterranean-DASH Intervention for Neurodegenerative Delay). This diet uses a combination of the Mediterranean diet and the DASH (Dietary Approaches to Stop Hypertension) diet as a basis but modifies them to place more emphasis on foods that have been linked by previous research to improved cognitive function and delayed decline.

The MIND Diet	
Include	Limit
Whole grains: 3 servings daily	Refined grains
Leafy green vegetables: Every day	Red meats: Fewer than four servings per week
Other vegetables: Every day	Butter and margarine: Less than 1 tablespoon daily
Nuts: Every day	Cheese: Less than one serving per week
Beans: Every other day	Pastries and sweets: Fewer than four servings per week
Berries: Every other day	Fried or fast food: Less than one serving per week
Poultry: At least twice per week	
Extra-virgin olive oil: Liberal use	
Wine: One glass per day	

The MIND trial followed 923 individuals aged 58 to 98 for an average of 4.5 years (in a range of 2 to 10 years). Diet was assessed using a 154-item guided questionnaire, and cognitive function was measured yearly using nineteen cognitive tests. Participants' diets were scored by how closely they matched up with recommendations for the Mediterranean, DASH, or MIND eating patterns. The key finding was that high adherence to any of these diets was associated with a reduced risk of cognitive decline. The MIND diet was judged the most effective overall, since even moderate adherence to it brought about a significant reduction in dementia risk. The researchers felt that the MIND diet was easier to follow because of its straightforward guidelines. I believe the guidelines for the Synergetic Diet are also easy to follow and have a bigger impact.

Anemia

Anemia can be due to excessive blood loss, excessive red blood cell destruction due to abnormal red blood cell shape, as in sickle-cell anemia, or, most commonly, deficient red blood cell production as a result of nutritional deficiencies. Although a deficiency of any of several vitamins and minerals can produce anemia, the most common cause is a deficiency of iron, vitamin B_{12}, or folic acid. Successful treatment of anemia requires accurate diagnosis based upon blood measurements.

The best food to eat for any type of anemia is iron- and B vitamin–rich calf's liver. Other foods rich in iron include leafy green vegetables, beans, blackstrap molasses, lean meats, almonds, and shellfish.

Tea, coffee, wheat bran, and egg yolks contain substances that inhibit iron absorption and should be avoided if iron absorption is a problem. Antacids and overuse of calcium supplements also decrease iron absorption.

When treating nutrition-related anemias, it is essential to supplement with the corresponding nutrient to address the deficiency. For example, supplementing with iron is the treatment for anemia due to iron deficiency, while vitamin B_{12} is used in treating anemia due to vitamin B_{12} deficiency.

Anxiety

Anxiety can be the result of both physical and psychological factors. While extreme stress can trigger anxiety, there are at least seven nutritional factors that may be responsible as well. Those include caffeine, sugar, food allergies, B vitamin deficiency, calcium or magnesium deficiency, and alcohol. Avoiding caffeine, sugar, and alcohol, as well as foods that trigger allergic reactions, often results in complete elimination of symptoms.

Boosting the intake of omega-3 fatty acids or taking a fish oil supplement to provide 3,000 mg of EPA+DHA per day can also be effective. Regular exercise is the best prescription for relieving stress and anxiety. Regular deep-breathing exercises and meditations can help as well.

Asthma

Many studies have indicated that food allergies play a role in asthma and its symptoms. Double-blind food challenges in children have shown that immediate-onset sensitivities are usually due (in decreasing order of frequency) to eggs, fish, shellfish, nuts, and peanuts; while foods most commonly associated with delayed-onset reactions include (in decreasing order of frequency) milk, chocolate, wheat, citrus, and food colorings. Elimination diets have been successful in treating asthma, particularly in infants and children (see Food Allergy, page 227).

Vitally important in the control of asthma is the elimination of food additives. Tartrazine (FD&C yellow dye No. 5), benzoates, sulfur dioxide, and, in particular, sulfites have been reported to cause asthma attacks in susceptible individuals. Tartrazine is found in most processed foods and even in vitamin preparations. It is estimated that 2 to 3 mg of sulfites are consumed each day by the average US citizen, while an additional 5 to 10 mg are ingested by regular wine and beer drinkers.

Switching to a vegan or vegetarian diet may also be of benefit. Asthma sufferers who followed a vegan diet (elimination of all animal products) experienced significant improvement. It is important to point out that although 71% of the patients responded within four months, one year of therapy was required before the 92% success level was reached. The diet excluded all meat, fish, eggs, and dairy products. Drinking water was limited to spring water (chlorinated tap water was specifically prohibited), and coffee, ordinary tea, chocolate, sugar, and salt were excluded. Herbs and spices were allowed, and water and herbal teas were allowed, up to 1½ liters per day. Vegetables eaten freely were lettuce, carrots, beets, onions, celery, cabbage, cauliflower, broccoli, nettles, cucumbers, radishes, Jerusalem artichokes, and all beans except soybeans and green peas. Potatoes were allowed in restricted amounts. A number of fruits were also allowed freely: blueberries, cloudberries, raspberries, strawberries, black currants, gooseberries, plums, and pears. Apples and citrus fruits were not allowed, and grains were either restricted or eliminated.

The beneficial effects of this dietary regime are likely related to three factors: (1) elimination of common food allergens, (2) altered fatty-acid metabolism, and (3) higher intake of dietary antioxidants. The compounds that contribute to the allergic and inflammatory reactions in asthma are derived primarily from arachidonic acid, a fatty acid found exclusively in animal products. In addition, several of the foods consumed (e.g., onions and berries) have exerted antiasthmatic effects in experimental studies. Onions are particularly beneficial.

My dietary recommendations for asthma are to eat a mostly vegetarian diet but include cold-water fish (salmon, mackerel, herring, etc.), which are rich in EPA+DHA. Increasing dietary fish intake and taking fish oil supplements have been shown to be quite helpful in reducing asthma severity.

Losing weight has also been shown to lead to significant decreases in asthma-related episodes of shortness of breath, increases in overall breathing capacity, and decreases in the need for medication to control symptoms.

Atherosclerosis, Heart Disease, and High Cholesterol Levels

Atherosclerosis is the process of the hardening of an artery due to the buildup of cholesterol-containing plaque. It is the underlying disease that is responsible for most heart attacks and strokes. The Synergetic Diet includes all the foods you should eat for a healthy heart and total well-being. My recommendations are to:

- Increase your intake of omega-3 oils by eating cold-water fatty fish, walnuts, and ground flaxseed. There is considerable evidence that people who consume a diet rich in omega-3 oils from either fish or other sources have a significantly reduced risk of developing atherosclerosis.

- Increase your intake of heart-healthy monounsaturated fats by eating more nuts and seeds and using monounsaturated oil such as extra-virgin olive, avocado, macadamia, or canola oil for cooking purposes.

- Eat seven or more servings daily of a combination of vegetables and fruits, especially green, orange, and yellow vegetables, berries, and citrus fruits.

- Consume flavonoid-rich superfoods such as cacao for their ability to improve endothelial cell function.

- Increase your intake of fiber; a diet high in fiber has been shown to be protective against atherosclerosis. Dietary fiber, particularly the soluble fiber found in legumes, ground flaxseed, fruits, and vegetables, is effective in lowering cholesterol levels.

- Limit your intake of refined carbohydrates (sugar and refined grains). They play a significant factor in the development of atherosclerosis. Sugar consumption elevates levels of the hormone insulin. Elevated insulin levels, in turn, are associated with increased cholesterol levels, triglyceride levels, blood pressure, and risk of death from cardiovascular disease.

The evidence overwhelmingly demonstrates that elevated cholesterol levels, especially of LDL cholesterol, greatly increase the risk of death due to a heart attack, stroke, or other cardiovascular disease. A wide array of dietary components has been shown to positively impact cholesterol levels; the best results are achieved with a combination of factors instead of just one. Again, the best strategy is to follow the broad-spectrum dietary approach represented by the Synergetic Diet. For example, while increasing the consumption of soy protein or eating oat bran can lower cholesterol levels, it is best to include a whole portfolio of cholesterol-lowering foods. This synergetic effect was observed in an analysis of twenty-seven clinical trials showing that when soy protein was used in conjunction with other dietary factors to lower cholesterol, significant reductions in total and LDL cholesterol were also included (–23.2 mg/dl, –21.7 mg/dl, and –3.3 mg/dl, respectively).

Here are some cholesterol-lowering foods to eat regularly:

- Garlic and onions, which can be effective in lowering blood lipids.

- Turmeric, capsicum, cinnamon, and ginger, to lower LDL cholesterol.

- Ground flaxseed, which has a multitude of health benefits, including lowering LDL cholesterol.

- Apples, which contain the soluble fiber pectin, which binds to cholesterol in the gut and escorts it out of the body. Clinical studies have shown that apple consumption can produce positive effects on both LDL ("bad") and HDL ("good") cholesterol levels. In one study, 160 women between the ages of 45 and 65 were divided into two groups. One group ate 75 grams of dried apple per day—about 2½ ounces— while the other ate the same amount of dried prunes. The women who ate apples experienced a 23% decrease in their LDL ("bad") cholesterol and an increase in their HDL ("good") cholesterol of 3% to 4%—a boost difficult to achieve with drugs or exercise. In addition, those who ate the apples, which contained about 240 calories, lost an average of about 3 pounds over the course of the year, probably because the apples helped satisfy their appetite with relatively few calories.

- Strawberries, blackberries, black raspberries, blueberries, cranberries, and red raspberries, which reduce the risk of cardiovascular disease by improving the plasma lipid profile, increasing plasma antioxidant activity, and improving the function of the cells that line blood vessels (endothelial cells). In one study, healthy volunteers ate 500 grams of strawberries (about 2½ cups) daily for 1 month. Strawberry consumption significantly reduced total cholesterol, low-density lipoprotein (LDL) cholesterol, and triglyceride levels (-8.78%, -13.72%, and -20.80%, respectively) compared with the baseline period.

Bladder Infection (Cystitis)

A bladder infection is one type of infection of the urinary system—kidneys, ureters, bladder, and urethra. To prevent bladder infections, drink more liquids in the form of pure water, herbal teas, cranberry juice, and fresh fruit and vegetable juices diluted with an equal amount of water. If you have a bladder infection, drink at least 64 ounces of liquids from this group, with at least half this amount being water, and at least 16 ounces unsweetened cranberry or blueberry juice. Avoid soft drinks, concentrated fruit drinks, coffee, and alcoholic beverages.

Cranberries have long been valued for their ability to reduce the risk of urinary tract infections (UTIs). This use became even more popular after a 1994 placebo-controlled study of 153 elderly women published in *The Journal of the American Medical Association* showed that cranberries help prevent UTIs. In this study, the women who drank the cranberry juice had fewer than half as many urinary infections—42% to be precise—as the control group, who received a placebo drink that contained no real cranberry juice. In this groundbreaking study, the dose of cranberry juice was 300 ml (about 1¼ cups), while in most of the later studies subjects drank about 16 ounces (2 cups) of cranberry juice each day.

Cranberry juice not only slightly acidifies the urine and contains an antibacterial agent called hippuric acid but, more important, has also been shown to reduce the ability of *E. coli* bacteria to adhere to the walls of the urinary tract. (For infection to occur, a pathogen must adhere to and penetrate the mucosal surface of the urinary tract walls. If *E. coli* cannot adhere, it's washed away and voided with the flow of urine.) Since 80% to 90% of urinary tract infections are caused by *E. coli*, cranberries provide significant protection against this common problem.

Canker Sores

Canker (mouth) sores are often associated with food allergies to milk products and wheat. Gluten, a grain protein, appears to be a causative factor for many individuals. Withdrawing gluten from the diet results in complete remission of recurrent canker sores in patients with gluten sensitivity.

The mouth and throat are often the first places where nutritional deficiency becomes visible because of the high turnover rate of the cells that line their surfaces. Several studies have shown nutrient deficiencies to be much more common among recurrent canker sore sufferers than in the general population, especially deficiencies of thiamin, folic acid, B_{12}, B_6, and iron. When the nutrient deficiencies were corrected, the majority of subjects with recurrent canker sores experienced complete remission.

Taking a high-potency multiple vitamin and mineral formula will ensure adequate intake of all nutrients linked to recurrent canker sores.

Cataracts

Cataracts are opaque white clouds that form on the normally transparent lens of the eyes, causing decreased vision in one or both eyes. They occur as a result of free-radical or oxidative damage to the protein structure of the lens.

Individuals with higher dietary intakes of antioxidant nutrients such as vitamins C and E, selenium, and carotenes have a much lower risk of developing cataracts. High-antioxidant foods such as leafy greens, yams, carrots, broccoli, and other brightly colored vegetables and fresh fruits provide these nutrients. The consumption of too much salt and saturated fat has been linked to cataract formation. It is also important to avoid fried and rancid foods and other sources of free radicals.

Particularly important in the prevention of cataracts may be increased glutathione levels. Glutathione is found in high concentrations in the lens, where it plays a vital role in maintaining a healthy lens. Glutathione functions as an antioxidant, maintains the structure of the lens proteins, acts in various enzyme systems, and participates in amino acid and mineral transport. Glutathione levels are diminished in people with virtually all forms of cataracts.

To raise glutathione levels, eat plenty of fresh and raw fruits and vegetables, as the glutathione content in these foods is substantially greater than that of their cooked counterparts.

Constipation

A low-fiber diet is often the cause of constipation. The combination of a high-fiber diet, plentiful fluid consumption, and exercise is an effective prescription in most cases of constipation. High levels of dietary fiber increase both the frequency and quantity of bowel movements, decrease the transit time of stools (the amount of time between consumption of a food and its elimination in the feces), the absorption of toxins from the stool, and appear to be a preventive factor in several diseases.

Consumption of cow's milk was determined to be the cause of constipation in roughly two-thirds of children with constipation, according to studies published in *The New England Journal of Medicine*.

Eating whole prunes or drinking 8 ounces of prune juice daily is an effective and gentle laxative. Prunes work faster and better than bulk fibers such as psyllium seed husks.

Depression

What if, in the treatment of depression, physicians quit relying on manipulating brain chemistry with drugs and focused instead on supporting brain chemistry through proper nutrition? A deficiency of any nutrient can alter brain function and lead to depression, anxiety, and other mental disorders, especially deficiencies of vitamin B_{12}, folic acid, other B vitamins, and omega-3 fatty acids.

Since the brain requires a constant supply of blood sugar to function properly, hypoglycemia (low blood sugar) should be avoided. Several studies have shown hypoglycemia to be common in depressed individuals. Just as in anxiety or insomnia, eliminating refined carbohydrates and caffeine from the diet helps some people manage their depression.

An analysis of a collection of scientific studies showed that a higher intake of fruits and vegetables is associated with a lower rate of depression. Some professionals view depression as an indication of low-grade inflammation within the brain. So dietary factors that reduce inflammation seem to have an ability to help prevent and treat depression. A study conducted at the University of Pittsburgh found that fewer college students were depressed or needed to take antidepressant drugs if they increased their intake of fish oil. To evaluate the effects of fish oil supplementation, the students were enrolled in a double-blind study. The subjects (mainly women) had significant depression, as evidenced by a score of greater than 10 on a standard diagnostic questionnaire (Beck Depression Inventory [BDI]) and were *not* taking an antidepressant drug. They were randomly assigned to a placebo (corn oil) or fish oil group (1.4 grams EPA+DHA daily). The BDI was completed prior to supplementation and again at day 21. The results demonstrated that there was a significant difference in depression status between groups. In those taking fish oils, 67% of the subjects no longer met the criteria for being depressed, while only 20% in the placebo group were no longer depressed. These results show that low-dosage fish oil supplementation is effective in boosting mood. These dosage levels of EPA+DHA can also be achieved by eating more cold-water fish.

Type 2 Diabetes

Dietary modification and treatment are fundamental to the successful control of diabetes. The dietary guidelines provided by the Synergetic Diet are especially important to follow in the prevention and treatment of diabetes. All simple, processed, and concentrated carbohydrates must be avoided. Low-glycemic-load foods should be eaten, particularly legumes, nuts, onions, and garlic. Saturated fats should be kept to a minimum. Weight loss, particularly a significant decrease in body fat percentage, is a prime objective in treating the majority of type 2 diabetics; it improves all aspects of diabetes and may result in a cure.

Several large population-based studies have shown that the higher the intake of fruits and vegetables, the better blood glucose levels are controlled and the lower the risk of developing type 2 diabetes. Several factors could explain this. Fruits and vegetables are good sources of fiber and have a high nutrient content and antioxidant content. Even something as simple as regular salad consumption is associated with a reduced risk of developing type 2 diabetes. Subjects reporting frequent consumption of a raw salad had a 50% reduced risk of developing type 2 diabetes compared with those who infrequently ate a salad.

Contrary to a popular misconception, fruit consumption can help fight against diabetes. Though fruit contains natural sugars, it also contains many compounds that promote health and reduce the risk of developing chronic diseases, including type 2 diabetes. The key in fruit consumption is to focus on low-glycemic-load choices, such as berries, and to limit consumption to one serving in any three-hour period to avoid stressing blood sugar control.

Diarrhea

Diarrhea is usually a mild, temporary event, but if it is ongoing, it may be the first indication of a serious underlying disease or infection. A physician should be consulted immediately if any of the following applies: diarrhea in a child under six years of age; severe or bloody diarrhea; diarrhea that lasts more than three days; and significant signs of dehydration (sunken eyes, severe dry mouth, strong body odor, etc.). Those with temporary diarrhea should:

- Avoid solid foods. During the acute phase of diarrhea, the focus should be on liquids.

- Replace water and electrolytes by consuming herbal teas, vegetable broths, fruit juices, and electrolyte replacement drinks. A naturopathic remedy is to sip a drink made of equal parts of sauerkraut juice and tomato juice.

- Avoid dairy products. Acute intestinal illnesses, such as viral or bacterial intestinal infections, frequently injure the cells that line the small intestine. This results in a temporary deficiency of lactase, the enzyme responsible for digesting the milk sugar (lactose) in dairy products. Avoid dairy products (with the possible exception of live-cultured yogurt) while experiencing diarrhea.

- Avoid food allergens. Food allergy is one of the most common causes of chronic diarrhea. The ingestion of an allergic food can result in the release of histamine and other allergic compounds from white blood cells known as mast cells that reside in the lining of the intestines. These allergic compounds can produce a powerful laxative effect.

- Consume pectin-rich fruits such as pears and apples, which may help solidify stools. Also, fresh blueberries have a long historical use in diarrhea.

- Consume carob. Carob comes from the pods of a Mediterranean tree. When the beans are dried and roasted, they have a cocoalike consistency and flavor. Clinical studies have confirmed the use of carob for treating diarrhea. Its beneficial effects are due primarily to its polyphenols and fiber compounds that become viscous in the gastrointestinal tract, helping to bind together watery stools. Carob can also bind to and inactivate toxins and inhibit the growth of bacteria. The usual dosage is at least 20 grams of carob powder stirred into water for adults; 15 grams of carob powder mixed with a little applesauce or mashed sweet potato provides a palatable, child-safe remedy for children 2 years and older.

Ear Infection (Otitis Media)

In acute otitis media, the middle ear, including the eardrum, becomes inflamed and infected. Ear infections are often preceded by an upper respiratory infection or allergy. A chronic ear infection is a constant swelling of the middle ear that can serve as a fertile breeding ground for an acute ear infection. Recurrent bouts of acute ear infections are responsible for more office visits by children to pediatricians than any other cause.

In some studies, elimination of food allergens has been shown to produce a dramatic effect in the treatment of chronic ear infections in more than 90% of children. Since it is usually not possible to determine the exact allergen during an acute attack, the most common allergenic foods should be eliminated from the diet: milk and other dairy products, eggs, wheat, corn, oranges, and peanut butter. Concentrated simple carbohydrates (sugar, honey, dried fruit, concentrated fruit juice, etc.) should also be eliminated since they inhibit the immune system.

Recurrent ear infections are strongly associated with bottle-feeding, while prolonged breastfeeding (minimum of six months) has a protective effect. Whether this is due to an allergy to formula or the protective effect of human milk against infection has not yet been determined, but most likely it is a combination of both. In addition, prolonged breastfeeding has been shown to prevent food allergies, particularly if the mother avoids sensitizing foods (those to which she is allergic) during pregnancy and lactation. Also of value is excluding the foods to which children are most commonly allergic: wheat, eggs, and dairy products, particularly during the first nine months.

Chewing gum sweetened with xylitol can be effective in treating ear infections. Xylitol is a natural sweetener derived mainly from birch and other hardwood trees. Two double-blind clinical trials have illustrated its ability to reduce acute ear infection incidence by 40%. In one study of 306 children in day care with recurrent acute otitis media, 157 children were given xylitol (8.4 grams per day) chewing gum and 149 children were given a sucrose control gum. During the two-month trial, at least one acute ear infection was experienced by 20.8% of the children who received sucrose, compared with only 12.1% of those receiving chewing gum containing xylitol. Significantly fewer antibiotics were prescribed for those receiving xylitol. In the second study, 857 healthy children were randomized to one of five treatment groups to receive control syrup, xylitol syrup, control chewing gum, xylitol gum, or xylitol lozenge. The daily dose of xylitol varied from 8.4 grams (chewing gum) to 10 grams (syrup). The study ran for three months. Although at least one event of otitis media was experienced by 41% of the 165 children who received the control syrup, only 29% of the 159 children receiving the xylitol syrup were affected. Likewise, the occurrence of otitis media decreased by 40% compared with control subjects in the children who received xylitol chewing gum and by 20% in the xylitol lozenge group. Thus the occurrence of acute ear infections during the follow-up period was significantly lower in those who received xylitol syrup or gum, and they required antimicrobials less often than did controls.

Eczema

Eczema is an allergic disorder of the skin. Elimination of food allergy is the primary goal in dealing with it. Although any food or food additive can trigger eczema, milk, eggs, and peanuts appear to be the most common food allergens. In one study, these three foods accounted for roughly 81% of all cases of childhood eczema. For more information on dealing with food allergies, see Food Allergy, page 227.

Patients with eczema also appear to have an essential fatty acid deficiency. This results in decreased synthesis of the anti-inflammatory prostaglandins. In addition, increasing the dietary intake of long-chain omega-3 oils, either by eating more fatty cold-water fish (mackerel, herring, and salmon) or taking fish oil supplements is of benefit.

Fibrocystic Breast Disease

Fibrocystic breast disease (FBD), also known as cystic mastitis, is a benign breast condition consisting of the presence of multiple cysts in the breast tissue. In addition to following the Synergetic Diet and focusing on consuming legumes, vegetables, fruits, nuts, and seeds, it is important to drink at least 48 ounces of water daily. These recommendations can help promote regular bowel movements. Women who have fewer than three bowel movements per week have a 4.5 times greater rate of developing FBD than women who have at least one bowel movement a day. This association is probably due to the bacterial flora in the large intestine transforming excreted steroids into toxic derivatives or allowing these excreted steroids to be reabsorbed.

Eliminating caffeine can also help prevent FBD. Population studies, experimental evidence, and clinical evaluations indicate a strong association between caffeine consumption and FBD. In one study, limiting consumption of coffee, tea, cola, chocolate, and caffeinated medications resulted in improvement in 97.5% of the forty-five women who completely abstained and in 75% of the twenty-eight women who limited their consumption. Drink herbal teas instead.

Food Allergy

A food allergy or sensitivity occurs when there is an adverse reaction to the ingestion of a food. The allergic reaction may or may not be mediated (controlled and influenced) by the immune system. The allergic reaction may be caused by a protein, starch, or other food component or by food additives (e.g., colorings, flavoring agents, or preservatives). Food allergies are associated with a multitude of symptoms and health conditions:

- Gastrointestinal: Canker sores, celiac disease, chronic diarrhea, duodenal ulcer, gastritis, irritable bowel syndrome, malabsorption, ulcerative colitis
- Genitourinary: Bed-wetting, chronic bladder infections, nephrosis
- Immune: Chronic infections, frequent ear infections
- Mental/emotional: Anxiety, depression, hyperactivity, inability to concentrate, insomnia, irritability, mental confusion, personality change, seizures
- Musculoskeletal: Bursitis, joint pain, lower back pain
- Respiratory: Asthma, chronic bronchitis, wheezing
- Skin: Acne, eczema, hives, itching, skin rash
- Other: Arrhythmia, edema, fainting, fatigue, headache, hypoglycemia, itchy nose or throat, migraines, sinusitis

An allergy elimination diet is valuable in identifying food allergies. In an allergy elimination diet, many commonly eaten foods are eliminated and replaced with either hypoallergenic foods and foods that are rarely eaten or special hypoallergenic formulas. The fewer the allergenic foods eaten, the greater the ease of establishing a diagnosis. The standard elimination diet includes lamb, chicken, potatoes, rice, bananas, apples, and cabbage-family vegetables (brussels sprouts, broccoli, etc.). Variations of this diet may be suitable.

The individual stays on the elimination diet for at least one week and up to one month. If the symptoms are related to food sensitivity, they will typically disappear by the fifth or sixth day of the diet. If the symptoms do not disappear, it is possible that a reaction to a food in the elimination diet is responsible. In that case, an even more restricted diet must be utilized.

After the elimination diet period, individual foods are reintroduced slowly. Methods range from reintroducing only a single food every two days to reintroducing a food every one or two meals. Usually, after the one-week "cleansing" period, the patient will develop an increased sensitivity to offending foods and discover which ones to avoid.

Reintroduction of allergenic foods will typically produce a more severe or recognizable symptom than before. A detailed food diary must be kept describing when foods are reintroduced and what symptoms appear upon reintroduction. It can be useful to track the wrist pulse during reintroduction, as pulse changes may occur when an allergenic food is consumed.

Gallstones

A low-fiber diet is one of the main causes of gallstones. Such a diet, which is typically high in refined carbohydrates and fat and low in fiber, leads to a reduction in the synthesis of bile acids by the liver, which in turn significantly reduces the solubility of the bile. A high intake of refined sugar is also a risk factor for gallstones.

The frequency of gallstones is two to four times as great in women as in men. Women are predisposed to gallstones because of either increased cholesterol synthesis or suppression of bile acids by estrogens. Pregnancy, use of oral contraceptives, or other causes of elevated estrogen levels greatly increase the incidence of gallstones. Obesity and constipation are also associated with a significant increase in risk.

Food allergies and intolerance have long been known to trigger gallbladder attacks. An interesting 1968 study revealed that 100% of a group of patients with gallstones were free from symptoms when they ate a basic elimination diet consisting of beef, rye, soybean, rice, cherries, peaches, apricots, beets, and spinach. Foods that induced symptoms of gallstones, in decreasing order of their occurrence, were eggs, pork, onions, fowl, milk, coffee, citrus fruits, corn, beans, and nuts. Adding eggs to the diet caused gallbladder attacks in

93% of the patients. However, despite these results, the role of food allergies in gallstone formation has not been looked at since that time.

A vegetarian diet has been shown to be protective against gallstone formation. While this may be a result of the increased fiber content of the vegetarian diet, other factors may be equally important. Animal proteins, such as casein from dairy products, have been shown to increase the formation of gallstones in animals, while vegetable proteins, such as soy, were shown to be preventive against gallstone formation.

Coffee (both regular and decaffeinated) induces gallbladder contractions, so if you have gallstones, avoid coffee until the stones are resolved.

Obesity causes an increased secretion of cholesterol in the bile as a result of increased cholesterol synthesis. It is important to recognize that during active weight reduction, bile cholesterol saturation initially increases. The secretion of all bile components is reduced during weight loss, but the secretion of bile acids decreases more than that of cholesterol. People on weight loss programs should support their liver function by eating high-fiber foods and drinking plenty of liquids. Consumption of 6 to 8 glasses of liquids each day is necessary to maintain the water content of bile. Pure water or fresh fruit and vegetable juices are the best ways to meet the body's liquid requirements. Once the weight is stabilized, bile acid output returns to normal levels, while cholesterol output remains low. The net effect of weight loss is a significant reduction in cholesterol saturation.

For prevention and treatment of gallstones, increase your intake of vegetables, fruits, and dietary fiber, especially gel-forming or mucilaginous fibers (found in flaxseed, oat bran, guar gum, pectin, etc.); reduce your consumption of saturated fats, cholesterol, sugar, and animal proteins; avoid all fried foods; and drink at least six 8-ounce glasses of water each day.

Gastroesophageal Reflux Disease (GERD) and Nonulcer Dyspepsia (NUD)

Gastroesophageal reflux disease (GERD) and nonulcer dyspepsia (NUD) are medical terms used to label indigestion and/or heartburn that is unrelated to an ulcer. The main symptoms of GERD are heartburn and/or upper abdominal pain.

GERD and NUD are most often caused by overeating. Other causes include obesity, smoking, chocolate and fried foods, and carbonated beverages, alcohol, and coffee. These factors either increase intra-abdominal pressure, thereby causing the gastric contents to flow upward, or decrease the tone of the esophageal sphincter. In most cases, eliminating or reducing the causative factor will relieve NUD and GERD. Decreasing portion sizes at mealtime may also help.

When one group of researchers looked at dietary factors to see if there was any link to GERD, what they found was that between-meals eating had the strongest association with GERD. A between-meals snack is thought to increase gastric distention in the upper stomach, as well as cause transient lower esophageal sphincter relaxation, triggering reflux. In contrast, fasting clears the stomach of food and reduces intra-abdominal pressure and reflux. Considering these factors, the researchers felt that two regular meals a day with only fluids in between would reduce reflux and lead to healing of the esophagus caused by repeated refluxes. In testing this simple regimen in a small number of patients, it was shown to eliminate symptoms of GERD in ten days. The researchers followed up with a pilot study in twenty patients of endoscopically diagnosed GERD. Results indicated that it benefited 100% of patients with mild GERD, 66% of patients with moderate GERD, and 33% of patients with severe GERD. These results indicate that this simple dietary recommendation can be effective in mild to moderate cases and should be used along with other natural approaches in more severe cases. Other remedies to consider:

• Carob powder can be quite helpful in relieving GERD symptoms. When ingested, carob's polyphenols and large sugar molecules form a gummy, viscous mix in the stomach, thereby blocking the reflux into the esophagus. The usual dosage for GERD is 1 to 2 tablespoons carob powder dissolved in 8 ounces of water before each meal.

- Lemons contain a substance known as d-limonene, with the highest content found in the peel and spongy white inner parts. A natural therapy for GERD is limonene, extracted from citrus fruit peel. Add 1 to 2 tablespoons fresh lemon juice to juices or salad dressings or squeeze on top of cooked vegetables.

- Fresh ginger offers relief from GERD as well. Add a ½-inch slice to fresh fruit or vegetable juices.

Gout

Gout is a common type of arthritis caused by an increased concentration of uric acid (the final breakdown product of purine, one of the units of DNA and RNA) in biological fluids. In gout, uric acid crystals are deposited in joints, tendons, kidneys, and other tissues, where they cause often painful inflammation and damage. The dietary treatment of gout involves the following guidelines.

- Avoid foods with high purine levels. These include organ meats, other meats, shellfish, yeast (brewer's and baker's), herring, sardines, mackerel, and anchovies. Intake of foods containing moderate levels of protein, including dried legumes, spinach, asparagus, fish, poultry, and mushrooms, should be reduced as well.

- Eliminate alcoholic beverages. Alcohol increases uric acid production by accelerating purine breakdown. It also reduces uric acid excretion by increasing lactate production, which impairs kidney function. Elimination of alcohol is all that is necessary to reduce uric acid levels and prevent gouty arthritis in many individuals.

- Lose weight. Obesity is associated with an increased rate of gout. Weight reduction in obese individuals significantly reduces serum uric acid levels. Weight reduction should involve the use of a high-fiber, low-fat diet to help manage the elevated cholesterol and triglyceride levels that are also common in obesity.

• Eat high fiber complex carbohydrates, such as legumes (moderate consumption), nuts, seeds, vegetables, and whole grains. Intake of refined carbohydrates, fructose, and saturated fat should be kept to a minimum. Simple sugars (refined sugar, honey, maple syrup, corn syrup, fructose, etc.) increase uric acid production, while saturated fats decrease uric acid excretion.

• Drink a lot of water. Liberal fluid intake keeps urine diluted and promotes the excretion of uric acid. Furthermore, diluting the urine reduces the risk of developing kidney stones. Drink at least 48 ounces of water each day.

• Eat cherries or drink cherry juice. Consuming 8 ounces of fresh or frozen unsweetened cherries per day has been shown to be effective in lowering uric acid levels and preventing attacks of gout. Add them to your smoothies or purchase cherry juice with no sugar added.

Hemorrhoids

Hemorrhoids are enlarged, painful veins in the anal/rectal area. A low-fiber diet that is high in refined foods contributes greatly to the development of hemorrhoids. Individuals who consume a low-fiber diet tend to strain more during bowel movements since their smaller, harder stools are more difficult to pass. This straining raises the pressure in the abdomen, which obstructs venous blood flow, increases pelvic congestion, and may significantly weaken the veins, causing hemorrhoids to form.

A high-fiber diet is the most important component in the prevention of hemorrhoids. A diet rich in vegetables, fruits, legumes, and grains promotes peristalsis, the normal rhythmic contractions of the intestines. Furthermore, many fiber components attract water and form a gelatinous mass that keeps the feces soft, bulky, and easy to pass. The net effect of a high-fiber diet is significantly less straining during defecation. The diet should also contain liberal amounts of flavonoid-rich foods, such as blackberries, citrus fruits, cherries, and blueberries, to strengthen the vein structures in the anus.

Herpes Simplex

Herpes simplex is a virus that is responsible for cold sores and genital herpes. The best approach to prevent recurrence is to focus on supporting the immune system. In this goal, it is especially important to avoid refined carbohydrates and food allergies. In addition, a diet high in the amino acid lysine and low in arginine can be an effective measure in preventing HSV infections, especially if used in conjunction with lysine supplementation (1,500 to 3,000 mg daily). This dietary approach arose from research showing that lysine has antiviral activity in test tube studies due to its ability to block arginine. HSV replication requires the manufacture of proteins rich in arginine, and arginine itself is suggested to be a stimulator of HSV replication. From a theoretical perspective, this approach should be effective, since in vitro studies have shown that HSV replication is dependent on adequate levels of arginine and low levels of lysine.

Foods high in arginine are chocolate, peanuts, seeds, and almonds and other nuts. Foods high in lysine include most vegetables, legumes, fish, turkey, and chicken.

High Blood Pressure

Although medical textbooks state that the cause is unknown in 95% of cases, hypertension is closely related to the health of an individual's arteries, lifestyle, and dietary factors. When the arteries become hard due to the buildup of plaque containing cholesterol, blood pressure rises. Just as in other degenerative diseases, the development of high blood pressure is closely related to lifestyle and dietary factors. Some of the important lifestyle factors that may cause high blood pressure include stress, lack of exercise, and smoking. Some of the dietary factors include obesity; high blood sodium-to-potassium ratio; a low-fiber, high-sugar diet; high saturated fat and low omega-3 fatty acid intake; and a diet low in calcium, magnesium, and vitamin C. These same factors are also known to impact the ability of the kidneys to regulate fluid volume and control blood pressure.

Two large studies have shown that diet can be effective in lowering blood pressure. These studies, called Dietary Approaches to Stop Hypertension (DASH), tested a diet rich in fruits, vegetables, and low-fat dairy foods and low in saturated and total fat. The DASH diet was also low in cholesterol, high in dietary fiber, potassium, calcium, and magnesium, and moderately high in protein.

The first study showed that a diet rich in fruits, vegetables, and low-fat dairy products can reduce blood pressure in the general population and people with hypertension. The original DASH diet did not require either sodium restriction or weight loss—the two traditional dietary tools to control blood pressure—to be effective. The second study from the DASH research group found that coupling the original DASH diet with sodium restriction was more effective than either dietary manipulation alone. The DASH diet produced a net blood pressure reduction of 11.4 and 5.5 mm Hg systolic and diastolic, respectively, in patients with hypertension. In the second trial, sodium intake was quantified at a "higher" intake of 3,300 mg per day; an "intermediate" intake of 2,400 mg per day; or a "lower" intake of 1,500 mg per day. Compared to the control diet, the DASH diet was associated with a significantly lower systolic blood pressure at each sodium level. The DASH diet with the lower sodium level led to a mean systolic blood pressure that was 7.1 mm Hg lower in participants without hypertension and 11.5 mm Hg lower in participants with hypertension. These results are clinically significant and indicate that a sodium intake below the recommended level of 2,400 mg daily can significantly and quickly lower blood pressure.

To lower blood pressure:

• Achieve and maintain ideal body weight. This is the most important recommendation for those with high blood pressure. Overweight people who lose even modest amounts of weight usually experience a reduction in blood pressure.

- Follow a diet high in potassium and low in sodium. Numerous studies have shown that sodium restriction alone does not improve blood pressure control in most people; it must be accompanied by a high potassium intake. Most Americans have a potassium-to-sodium ratio of less than 1:2, meaning they ingest twice as much sodium as potassium. Researchers recommend a dietary potassium-to-sodium ratio of greater than 5:1 to maintain health. The easiest way to decrease sodium intake is to avoid prepared foods and table salt. Replace with a potassium chloride salt substitute, such as NoSalt and Nu-Salt. Boost potassium levels by eating more fruits, vegetables, whole grains, and legumes.

- Drink beet juice; eat garlic and onions and nuts and seeds or their oils for their essential fatty acid content, cold-water fish or fish oil products with a high concentration of EPA and DHA, leafy green vegetables as a rich source of calcium and magnesium, legumes for their fiber, and foods rich in vitamin C such as broccoli and citrus fruits.

- In a study conducted at the St. Boniface Hospital Research Centre in Winnipeg, Canada, the effects of daily ingestion of ground flaxseed on systolic blood pressure (SBP) and diastolic blood pressure (DBP) in patients with peripheral artery disease was studied. Though individuals with normal blood pressure showed no effect over six months of flaxseed ingestion (2 tablespoons daily), those patients who entered the trial with a SBP of ≥140 mm Hg at baseline obtained an average reduction of 15 mm Hg in SBP and 7 mm Hg in DBP. In other words, this major antihypertensive effect was achieved selectively in hypertensive patients.

- Celery is another interesting food when it comes to lowering blood pressure. A celery seed extract standardized to contain 85% 3-n-butylphthalide (NBP) has been shown to help improve blood pressure control. NBP is a compound that is unique to celery and is responsible for its characteristic flavor and aroma. It was discovered as the active component of celery in response to investigations by researchers seeking to explain some of the traditional effects of celery, including reduction of blood pressure and relief of joint pain. The dosage of the extract is 75 to 150 mg twice daily. This would translate to six to twelve ribs of celery, too much to eat whole but good for juicing.

• Two clinical studies have shown grape seed extract (standardized to contain 95% procyanidolic oligomers) to normalize high blood pressure in patients with initial blood pressure in the range of 150/95 mm Hg. The dosage was 300 mg daily. This amount can be achieved through dietary means by focusing on proanthocyanidin-rich foods. A study conducted at Florida State University included forty-eight postmenopausal women with mild hypertension enrolled to evaluate the effects of daily blueberry consumption for eight weeks. The women were randomly assigned to receive either 22 grams of freeze-dried blueberry powder or 22 grams of control powder daily, 22 grams of freeze-dried blueberry powder is equal to approximately 1 cup of fresh blueberries, an attainable dosage to consume on a daily basis. After eight weeks, systolic blood pressure and diastolic blood pressure (131 mm Hg and 75 mm Hg, respectively) were significantly lower than the baseline levels (138 mm Hg, 80 mm Hg) among the women who received blueberry powder, whereas there were no changes in the group receiving the control powder. Blueberry consumption was also associated with improved elasticity within the arteries.

Hives (Urticaria)

Hives (urticaria) is an allergic reaction in the skin characterized by itchy white or pink welts or large bumps surrounded with redness. Food allergy is the most common cause of hives, especially in chronic cases. The foods that most commonly trigger hives are milk, eggs, chicken, cured meat, alcoholic beverages, cheese, chocolate, citrus fruits, shellfish, and nuts. Food additives that trigger hives include colorants (azo dyes), flavorings (salicylates), artificial sweeteners (aspartame), preservatives (benzoates, nitrites, sorbic acid), antioxidants (hydroxytoluene, sulfite, gallate), and emulsifiers/stabilizers (polysorbates, vegetable gums). Numerous clinical studies demonstrate that diets free of food allergens and/or food additives typically produce significant reductions in roughly 50% to 75% of people with chronic hives.

- The best dietary recommendation is an allergy elimination diet, or at the least, a diet that excludes all food allergen and all food additives. The strictest allergy elimination diet allows only water, lamb, rice, pears, and vegetables for at least one week. If the hives are related to a food allergy or food additives, they will typically disappear by the fifth or sixth day of the diet. After one week, individual foods are reintroduced at a rate of one new food every three days. Reintroduction of offending foods will typically produce a more severe or recognizable symptom than before.

Hypoglycemia

Hypoglycemia is low blood sugar. Dietary carbohydrates play a central role in the cause, prevention, and treatment of hypoglycemia. The body quickly absorbs simple carbohydrates, or sugars, resulting in a rapid elevation in blood sugar level; this stimulates a corresponding excessive elevation in serum insulin levels, which can then lead to hypoglycemia.

All simple, processed, and concentrated carbohydrates and high-glycemic-load foods must be avoided. Avoid alcoholic drinks, as their consumption severely stresses blood sugar control and is often a contributing factor to hypoglycemia. Alcohol induces reactive hypoglycemia by interfering with normal glucose utilization and increasing the secretion of insulin. The resultant drop in blood sugar produces a craving for food, particularly foods that quickly elevate blood sugar levels, as well as a craving for more alcohol. The increased sugar consumption aggravates the reactive hypoglycemia, particularly in the presence of more alcohol.

A balanced diet with regular meals is recommended.

Immune Support

Consistent with good health, optimal immune function requires a healthy diet that (1) is rich in whole, natural foods, such as fruits, vegetables, grains, beans, seeds, and nuts, (2) is low in fats and refined sugars, and (3) contains adequate, but not excessive, amounts of protein. For optimal immune function, drink five or six 8-ounce glasses of water per day, take a basic multivitamin-multimineral supplement, engage in a regular exercise program of at least thirty minutes of aerobic exercise and five to ten minutes of stretching daily, perform daily deep-breathing and relaxation exercises (meditation, prayer, etc.), take time each day to play and enjoy family and friends, and get at least six to eight uninterrupted hours of sleep each night.

One of the food components most damaging to our immune system is sugar. In one study, the ingestion of 100 grams (roughly 3½ ounces) of carbohydrate such as glucose, fructose, sucrose, honey, or pasteurized orange juice all significantly reduced the ability of white blood cells (neutrophils) to engulf and destroy bacteria. In contrast, the ingestion of 100 grams of starch (a complex carbohydrate) had no effect. These effects started less than thirty minutes after ingestion and lasted for more than five hours. Typically, there was at least a 50% reduction in neutrophil activity two hours after ingestion. Since neutrophils constitute 60% to 70% of the total circulating white blood cells, impairment of their activity leads to depressed immunity.

In addition, ingestion of 75 grams of glucose has been shown to depress lymphocyte activity. Other parameters of immune function are also undoubtedly affected by sugar consumption. It has been suggested that the ill effects of high glucose levels are a result of competition between blood glucose and vitamin C for membrane transport sites into the white blood cells. This is based on evidence that vitamin C and glucose appear to have opposite effects on immune function and the fact that both require insulin for membrane transport into many tissues.

Considering that the average American consumes 150 grams of sucrose, plus other refined simple sugars, each day, the inescapable conclusion is that most Americans have chronically depressed immune systems. It is clear, particularly during an infection or chronic illness, that the consumption of refined sugars is harmful to immune function. To enhance your immune function:

- Eat foods loaded with carotenes: carrots, sweet potatoes, dark leafy greens, and tomatoes. Many of the immune-enhancing effects of carotenes, as well as other antioxidants, are due to their ability to protect the main organ of the immune system, the thymus gland, from damage.

- Consume other foods that are important for proper immune function, including cabbage-family vegetables, flavonoid-rich berries, garlic, onions, and lemons.

Insomnia

Insomnia is a sleep disorder. Some people have trouble falling asleep, while others wake up during the night and find it impossible to go back to sleep. Coffee, as well as less obvious caffeine sources such as soft drinks, chocolate, coffee-flavored ice cream, hot cocoa, and tea must all be eliminated. Even small amounts of caffeine, such as those found in decaffeinated coffee or chocolate, may be enough to cause insomnia in some people.

Foods high in tryptophan, such as turkey, milk, cottage cheese, chicken, eggs, soybeans, tofu, and nuts, especially almonds, may help promote sleep. In the brain, tryptophan is converted to serotonin and melatonin, which are natural sleep-inducing compounds.

If you are on a blood sugar roller coaster, it may be causing you to suffer from sleep maintenance insomnia. This means that you fall asleep but awaken three to five hours later, and have a difficult time getting back to sleep. Follow a low-glycemic diet, avoid alcohol, and take PGX before all major meals.

Irritable Bowel Syndrome (IBS)

IBS is characterized by some combination of the following symptoms: abdominal pain or distension; altered bowel function, constipation, or diarrhea; hypersecretion of colonic mucus; dyspeptic symptoms (flatulence, nausea, anorexia); and varying degrees of anxiety or depression.

There appear to be four main causes of IBS: stress, insufficient intake of dietary fiber, food allergies, and foods that contain too much sugar. Stress increases the motility (the rhythmic contractions of the intestine that propel food through the digestive tract) of the colon and leads to abdominal pain and irregular bowel function.

Food allergy as a cause of IBS has been recognized since the early 1900s. Studies have shown approximately two-thirds of patients with IBS have at least one food allergy and in some cases multiple allergies. The most common allergens are dairy products (40% to 44%) and grains (40% to 60%). Many patients have noted marked clinical improvement when eliminating these foods. Meals high in refined sugar can contribute to IBS by decreasing intestinal motility. When blood sugar levels rise too rapidly, the normal rhythmic contractions of the gastrointestinal tract slow down and in some areas may stop altogether. A diet high in refined sugar may be the key factor in why IBS is far more common in the United States than in other countries.

- Ginger is an excellent carminative (a substance that promotes the elimination of intestinal gas) and intestinal spasmolytic (a substance that relaxes and soothes the intestinal tract). Add a ¼-inch slice when juicing fresh fruits or vegetables. For a soothing juice, juice ¼-inch slice of ginger, ½ handful fresh peppermint or spearmint, ½ small fennel bulb, and 1 apple, cut into wedges.

Kidney Stones

Kidney stones are pieces of solid material that become stuck in the urinary tract. They can be quite painful. They are most often composed of calcium oxalate crystals and are associated with low fiber, highly refined carbohydrates, high alcohol consumption, large amounts of animal protein, and high fat intake. The best ways to protect against kidney stones are to:

- Increase your intake of fiber, complex carbohydrates, and green leafy vegetables, and decrease your intake of simple carbohydrates. Increase your intake of high-magnesium-to-calcium-ratio foods (barley, bran, corn, buckwheat, rye, soy, oats, brown rice, avocado, bananas, cashews, coconut, peanuts, sesame seeds, lima beans, potatoes). If oxalate stones are present, reduce your intake of oxalate-containing foods (e.g., black tea, cocoa, spinach, rhubarb).

- Eat your fruits and vegetables. Studies have shown that, even among meat eaters, those who ate higher amounts of fresh fruits and vegetables had a lower incidence of kidney stones. The simple change from white to whole wheat bread has resulted in lowering urinary calcium levels.

- Avoid excess sugar consumption. The ingestion of sucrose and other simple sugars causes an exaggerated increase in the urinary calcium oxalate content in approximately 70% of people with recurrent kidney stones.

- Avoid excess salt consumption. Salt contributes to kidney stones by increasing calcium excretion. People who tend to form kidney stones have an even greater increase in urinary calcium with an increase in salt intake.

- Drink more water. Increasing the urine volume results in a decrease in kidney stone formation. Numerous clinical trials have found that consumption of 2 or more liters of water per day or increasing fluid intake to achieve a urine output of 2.5 liters or more per day lowers the long-term risk of kidney stone recurrence by approximately 60%.

Macular Degeneration

The macula is the area of the retina where images are focused. It is the portion of the eye responsible for fine vision. Age-related macular degeneration (ARMD) is the leading cause of severe visual loss in the United States in people aged 55 and older. The major risk factors for macular degeneration are smoking, aging, atherosclerosis (hardening of the arteries), and high blood pressure.

A diet rich in fruits and vegetables is associated with a lowered risk of developing ARMD. Presumably, this protection is the result of increased intake of antioxidant vitamins and minerals. However, various "nonessential" food components, including carotenes such as lutein, zeaxanthin, and lycopene, along with flavonoids, are proving to be even more significant in protecting against ARMD than traditional nutritional antioxidants such as vitamin C, vitamin E, and selenium.

The macula, especially the central portion (the fovea), owes its yellow color to its high concentration of lutein and zeaxanthin. These yellow carotenes function to prevent oxidative damage to the area of the retina responsible for fine vision and play a central role in protecting against the development of macular degeneration.

To help prevent ARMD, eat plenty of dark, leafy greens and vibrantly colored vegetables.

Menopause

Menopause is defined as occurring twelve months after the last menstrual period. Due to lower estrogen levels, women are no longer able to bear children. As estrogen levels change, uncomfortable symptoms may include hot flashes, night sweats, headaches, weight gain, interrupted sleep, and many more. To help alleviate the symptoms of menopause:

- Increase your intake of plant foods, especially those high in phytoestrogens, while reducing the amount of animal foods you consume. Phytoestrogens are plant compounds that are capable of binding to estrogen receptors. Foods high in phytoestrogens include soy, flaxseed, nuts, whole grains, apples, fennel, celery, parsley, and alfalfa. A high intake of phytoestrogens is thought to explain why hot flashes and other menopausal symptoms are less common in populations that consume a predominantly plant-based diet. Increasing the intake of dietary phytoestrogens helps decrease hot flashes, increase the maturation of vaginal cells, and inhibit osteoporosis. In addition, a diet rich in phytoestrogens results in a decreased frequency of breast, colon, and prostate cancer.

- Consume ground flaxseed (2 to 3 tablespoons daily) and soy foods. Clinical studies have shown flaxseed intake, soy foods, and soy supplements providing isoflavones to be effective in relieving hot flashes and promoting bone health. Maximum benefit is achieved by consuming 45 to 90 mg of soy isoflavones daily.

- Consume procyanidin-rich foods such as grapes with seeds (eat the seeds), berries, nuts, seeds, and beans. A double-blind study with 30 mg of pine bark extract (Pycnogenol) rich in procyanidins taken twice per day was found to significantly improve all symptoms and produced a decrease in severity of all menopausal symptoms by 56% after twelve weeks of treatment. Pycnogenol was found to be especially effective in improving hot flashes and insomnia/sleep problems, the two most common and bothersome symptoms of menopause. What was particularly interesting about this study was how effective this relatively low daily dose of Pycnogenol was. Typically, for many therapeutic indications, the daily dosage has been in the range of 50 to 150 mg.

Migraine Headaches

Food allergy or sensitivity plays a primary role in some cases of migraine headache. Many double-blind, placebo-controlled studies have demonstrated that the detection and removal of allergenic foods eliminate or greatly reduce migraine symptoms in the majority of patients. Food allergy/intolerance induces a migraine attack largely as a result of platelets releasing serotonin and histamine. In addition, foods such as chocolate, cheese, beer, and wine contain histamine and/or other compounds that can trigger migraines in sensitive individuals by causing blood vessels to expand. Red wine is much more likely than white wine to cause a headache because it contains higher levels of phenols and 20 to 200 times as much histamine. Hypoglycemia can also trigger a migraine.

Ginger can be effective in preventing migraine attacks. A team of Iranian neurologists compared ginger and sumatriptan, the standard drug used to treat migraines in a double-blind study of one hundred men and women who suffered from migraines for an average of seven years. Some were given a box of five caplets containing their test medication: a 250 mg caplet of dried ginger powder or an identical-looking caplet containing 50 mg of sumatriptan in a double-blind fashion. The subjects were instructed to take a caplet at the onset of a migraine.

For each headache, the participants recorded when the headache began, headache severity before taking the medication, and degree of pain relief at 30, 60, 90, and 120 minutes as well as twenty-four hours after taking it. The results showed that ginger was equally as effective as sumatriptan, achieving 90% relief within two hours after ingestion. A small percentage (4%) of those who took the ginger caplets experienced minor digestive symptoms, while 20% of the subjects taking sumatriptan reported dizziness, drowsiness, or heartburn.

- To counteract a migraine, add a ¼-inch slice to juice when you feel the migraine beginning. You can also make ginger ale by stirring grated ginger into sparkling water.

Obesity

There are literally hundreds of diets and diet programs that claim to be the answer to obesity. One of the best things you can do to lose weight is to eat more dietary fiber. An increased intake of dietary fiber or fiber supplementation has been shown to enhance blood sugar control, decrease insulin levels, and reduce the number of calories absorbed by the body. The best fiber sources for promoting weight loss are those that are rich in water-soluble fibers, such as PGX, glucomannan (from konjac root), psyllium, guar gum, defatted fenugreek seed powder or fiber, seaweed fiber (alginate, carrageenan), and pectin.

When taken with water before meals, these fiber sources bind to the water in the stomach and small intestine to form a gelatinous, viscous mass that not only slows the absorption of glucose but induces a sense of fullness and reduces the absorption of calories.

It is important to maintain muscle mass during weight loss. Muscle mass is the body's primary fat-burning furnace. A muscle cell burns as much as fifteen times as many calories per day as a fat cell. Muscle mass is the primary factor that determines how quickly a person will lose weight, and low muscle mass is a primary reason why many people hit a plateau at some point during a weight-loss program.

To help maintain muscle mass during weight loss, be sure to exercise and include weight training exercises. I also recommend adding whey protein to your diet.

Osteoarthritis

Osteoarthritis (also known as degenerative joint disease) is a form of arthritis (inflammation of a joint) caused by the degeneration of cartilage. Cartilage's gel-like structure provides protection to the ends of bones by acting as a shock absorber. When the cartilage in a joint wears away, the bone literally rubs against the adjoining bone, leading to pain, deformity, inflammation, and limitation of motion. The most important things to do to reduce the probability of developing osteoarthritis or to alleviate it are to:

Multiple Sclerosis

In 1948, Dr. Roy Swank, professor of neurology at the University of Orego Medical School, started providing convincing evidence that a diet low in sa urated fats, maintained over a long period of time, tends to retard the disease process of multiple sclerosis (MS) and reduce the number of attacks. He rec- ommended:

- A saturated fat intake of no more than 10 grams per day
- A daily intake of 40 to 50 grams of polyunsaturated oils per day (marga- rine, shortening, and hydrogenated oils are not allowed)
- At least 1 teaspoon cod liver oil per day
- Consumption of cold-water fish three or more times per week

The Swank diet was originally thought to help patients with MS by over- coming essential fatty acids deficiency. It is now thought that the beneficial effects are probably a result of (1) a decrease in platelet aggregation, (2) a decrease in autoimmune response, and (3) normalization of the deficiency of essential fatty acids.

A high intake of saturated fatty acids and animal fat is linked to the devel- opment of MS. Consumption of saturated fats increases the requirements for the essential fatty acids, creating a relative deficiency state. Making matters worse is that individuals with MS are also thought to have a defect in essential fatty acid absorption and/or transport, which results in a functional deficiency state. Without essential fatty acids, the nerves' myelin sheath does not form or function properly.

Food allergy, in particular the consumption of two common allergens, gluten and milk, has been implicated in the progression of MS. Though there is no solid clinical evidence that a gluten-free or allergy elimination diet is beneficial in the management of MS, it certainly is healthful to eliminate food allergens (as long as other dietary measures are also included, for example, the Swank diet); there is anecdotal evidence that specific individuals have been helped.

- Achieve a normal body weight. Being overweight creates increased stress on weight-bearing joints affected with osteoarthritis.

- Eat a diet that is rich in nuts, seeds, fruits, and vegetables. The natural compounds they contain can protect against cellular damage, including damage to the joints. Foods especially beneficial in osteoarthritis are flavonoid-rich fruits such as cherries, blueberries, and blackberries.

- Consume nuts and seeds. Consuming 40 grams of sesame seeds per day has been shown to reduce inflammation, reduce pain, and improve joint function in patients with osteoarthritis. Consumption of other nuts and seeds may offer similar benefits.

- Eat sulfur-rich foods such as garlic, onions, brussels sprouts, and cabbage. The sulfur content in the fingernails of arthritis sufferers is lower than that of subjects without arthritis.

- Consume ginger, which may be helpful because of its anti-inflammatory effects. In a six-week study of 261 patients with knee osteoarthritis, 63% of those who consumed ginger found some relief versus 50% of the placebo users. Those in the ginger group resorted to acetaminophen less frequently and had a reduction in knee pain on standing and after walking.

- Consider avoiding foods in the nightshade family. It appears that in genetically susceptible individuals, long-term, low-level consumption of the alkaloids found in tomatoes, potatoes, eggplant, and peppers can worsen osteoarthritis. It is thought that these alkaloids inhibit normal collagen repair in the joints or promote the inflammatory degeneration of the joint. Although this hypothesis remains to be proved, a diet free of nightshade-family fruits and vegetables may provide some benefit to certain individuals and is certainly worth a try.

Osteoporosis

Osteoporosis literally means "porous bone." Though many people erroneously consider osteoporosis to be the result of the loss of calcium and other bone minerals, it involves a loss of both the mineral (inorganic) and nonmineral (organic matrix, composed primarily of protein) components of bone. Bone is dynamic living tissue that is constantly being broken down and rebuilt. Osteoporosis occurs when there is more bone breaking down than being formed.

Normal bone metabolism is dependent on an intricate interplay of many nutritional, lifestyle, and hormonal factors. Poor bone health is most common in postmenopausal Asian and Caucasian women. Other risk factors include a family history of osteoporosis; physical inactivity; short stature, low body mass, and/or small bones; and never having been pregnant.

Although nutritional factors are important, physical exercise, consisting of one hour of moderate activity (walking, weight lifting, dancing, etc.) three times a week, has been shown to prevent bone loss and increase bone mass in postmenopausal women.

A high-protein diet is associated with increased excretion of calcium in the urine as well as increased risk of developing osteoporosis. Raising the daily protein intake from 47 to 142 grams doubles the excretion of calcium in the urine. Too little protein, however, is also associated with poor bone health.

A diet high in salt or acid ash also causes calcium removal from bones and increases calcium loss in the urine. Therefore, it is important to avoid salt and follow an alkaline-based diet. An alkaline diet is one that focuses on vegetables, fruits, nuts, and legumes while avoiding overconsumption of meat and dairy. Soft drinks containing phosphates (phosphoric acid) should certainly be avoided.

Refined-sugar intake also increases the loss of calcium from the bones via the blood through the urine. Calcium is then pulled from the bones to maintain blood calcium levels, as foods containing refined sugar do not contain calcium. Some things to be aware of regarding osteoporosis:

- Leafy green vegetables (kale, collard greens, parsley, lettuce, etc.), as well as green tea, provide significant protection against osteoporosis.

These foods are a rich source of a broad range of vitamins and minerals that are important to maintaining healthy bones, including calcium, vitamin K_1, and boron. Vitamin K_1 is the form of vitamin K that is found in plants. One function of vitamin K_1 is to convert inactive osteocalcin to its active form. Osteocalcin is an important protein; its role is to anchor calcium molecules within the bone. The K_2 form is even more effective in activating osteocalcin. Fermented forms of soy, such as natto, are especially rich sources of vitamin K_2. Supplementing with 180 mcg per day has been shown to significantly improve bone health and density.

• Soy foods have the potential to favorably affect bone metabolism due to the presence of isoflavones. Numerous studies have shown that soy consumption is associated with greater bone density. The benefits are seen when the intake of soy isoflavones is at least 90 mg per day. Studies of lower levels of intake have consistently failed to show any real benefit to bone health.

• Prunes have been shown to help offset a woman's significantly increased risk for accelerated bone loss during the first three to five years after menopause. When fifty-eight postmenopausal women ate about twelve prunes each day for three months, they were found to have higher blood levels of enzymes and growth factors that indicate bone formation than women who did not consume prunes. Plus, none of the women suffered any adverse gastrointestinal side effects. Prunes' beneficial effects on bone formation may be due to their high concentration of phenolic compounds, which act as antioxidants to curb bone loss. They also provide a good supply of boron, a trace mineral integral to bone metabolism that is thought to play an important role in the prevention of osteoporosis. A single serving (¼ cup or 100 grams) of prunes provides 2 to 3 mg of boron.

Prostate Enlargement (Benign Prostatic Hyperplasia)

Benign (nonmalignant) enlargement of the prostate gland is known medically as benign prostatic hyperplasia, or BPH for short. Because an enlarged prostate can pinch off the flow of urine, BPH is characterized by symptoms of bladder obstruction, such as increased urinary frequency, nighttime awakening to empty the bladder, and reduced force and caliber (flow speed) of urination.

Current estimates are that BPH affects more than 50% of men during their lifetime. The frequency increases with advancing age, from approximately 5% to 10% at age 30 to more than 90% in men over 85 years of age.

Diet plays a critical role in the health of the prostate. The most important dietary guidelines to follow are:

- Focus on whole, unprocessed foods (whole grains, legumes, vegetables, fruits, nuts, and seeds). Eat ¼ cup of raw sunflower seeds or pumpkin seeds each day, and consume soy foods and lycopene-rich vegetables such as tomatoes, spinach, kale, mangoes, broccoli, and berries regularly.

- Reduce your intake of alcohol (especially beer), caffeine, and sugar.

- Eat organic foods to avoid pesticides and other contaminants (e.g., dioxin, polyhalogenated biphenyls, hexachlorobenzene, and dibenzofurans), which may have contributed to the increased occurrence of BPH in the last few decades. BPH is just one of many health problems that may be due to these toxic substances. A diet rich in organic fruits, vegetables, legumes, nuts, and seeds may provide some protection due to the presence of many phytochemicals.

- Drink cranberry juice, which may help relieve symptoms due to inflammation of the prostate. Forty-two men with chronic nonbacterial prostatitis received either 1,500 mg of powdered cranberries per day for six months or no cranberry powder at all. At the end of the study, the cranberry-powder group experienced significant improvements in Interna-

tional Prostate Symptom Score (IPSS), quality of life, and urine flow
and other voiding parameters, but the control group did not. The mean
IPSS declined by 4.48 points in the cranberry group compared with an
increase of 1.43 in the control group.

- Eat tomatoes. Lycopene, the red pigment in tomatoes, has shown benefits in improving prostate health and protecting against the development
  of prostate cancer. Harvard University researchers discovered that men
  who consumed the highest levels of lycopene (6.5 mg per day) in their
  diet showed a 21% decreased risk of prostate cancer compared with
  those consuming the lowest levels. Men who ate two or more servings of
  tomato sauce each week were 23% less likely to develop prostate cancer
  during the twenty-two years of the study than men who ate less than one
  serving of tomato sauce each month.

To determine the effect of typical servings of commercially available
tomato products on blood and prostate lycopene concentrations, men scheduled to undergo removal of their prostate glands due to cancer were randomized either to a lycopene-restricted control group (<5 mg of lycopene per day)
or to groups providing 25 to 35 mg of lycopene per day from the following
tomato products: tomato soup (2 to 2¾ cups prepared per day); tomato sauce
(5 to 7 ounces per day); or vegetable juice (11 to 16.5 fluid ounces per day).

Tomato soup, sauce, and juice consumption significantly increased the
subjects' plasma lycopene concentration by 66%, 71%, and 59%, respectively,
while the controls consuming the lycopene-restricted diet showed a decline in
plasma lycopene concentration of 24%. The end-of-study prostate lycopene
concentration was 3.5-, 3.6-, and 2.2-fold higher in the tomato soup, sauce,
and juice consumers, respectively. These results indicate that the tomato
products at the levels consumed were all effective at boosting lycopene levels
in the prostate.

Interestingly, in the tomato products, 80% to 90% of the lycopene was in
the trans (linear) configuration, while in the blood and prostate isomers, 47%
and 80%, respectively, were in the cis (bent) form. This difference demonstrates a shift toward cis accumulation and perhaps a preference for the cis iso-

mer over the trans. You can increase the cis form in tomato paste by heating it at 260°F for at least forty minutes. This will increase the amount of cis isomers ninefold. Add 1 tablespoon extra-virgin olive oil to further increase lycopene absorption.

Psoriasis

Psoriasis is a skin disorder characterized by the appearance of plaquelike, silvery scale lesions caused by a pileup of skin cells that have replicated too rapidly. In addition to affecting the skin, psoriasis can cause an inflammatory form of arthritis and affect the nails.

The key dietary recommendations are to limit the consumption of sugar while increasing the intake of high-fiber foods such as vegetables, legumes, fruits, and whole grains. Dietary fiber helps bind gut-derived toxins that can be absorbed and trigger psoriasis. However, it appears that many psoriasis patients do well by avoiding sources of gluten, like wheat. In fact, an allergy elimination diet can often help psoriasis. Follow the recommendations given under Food Allergy, page 227. In addition:

- Avoid alcohol, since it is known to worsen psoriasis by increasing the absorption of toxins from the gut that can stimulate psoriasis.

- Eat the right types of fats to reduce inflammation. Limit your consumption of meat and animal fats, and eat more cold-water fish. In the skin of individuals who have psoriasis, there is an increased production of inflammatory compounds produced from the animal fat arachidonic acid. Since arachidonic acid is found only in animal tissues, limit your intake of animal products, particularly meat, animal fats, and dairy products. At the same time, it is important to increase your intake of the long-chain omega-3 fatty acids from fish because of their favorable effects on reducing inflammation. Fish oil supplements rich in eicosapentaenoic acid (EPA) and docosahexaenoic acid (DHA) have also been shown to be helpful in improving psoriasis. The dosage used in double-blind clinical studies has typically provided 1.8 grams of EPA and 1.2 grams of DHA per day for a total of 3 grams of EPA+DHA.

- Increase your intake of procyanidin-rich foods, such as grapes with seeds (eat the seeds), berries, nuts, seeds, and beans. A double-blind study with pine bark extract (Pycnogenol) showed good results in controlling psoriasis. In the study, seventy-three patients with moderate to severe plaque psoriasis received "standard drug management" alone or with Pycnogenol at a dosage of 150 mg per day (50 mg three times daily). Over twelve weeks, the addition of Pycnogenol was shown to:

  - Significantly decrease the area of skin affected by psoriasis in all body regions (Pycnogenol 20%; standard management [SM] 8%)
  - Significantly reduce redness (Pycnogenol 44%; SM 28%), skin hardening (Pycnogenol 45%; SM 21%) and flaking (Pycnogenol 45%; SM 16%) of body area affected by psoriasis
  - Significantly increase water and oil/lipids content in all areas of the skin
  - Significantly reduce the need for standard management drugs
  - Significantly reduce oxidative stress
  - Significantly decrease the cost of treatment (on average by 36.4% in comparison with the standard management) and reduce the number of side effects reported with other treatments

Rheumatoid Arthritis

Rheumatoid arthritis (RA) is a chronic inflammatory condition that affects the entire body, but especially the hands, feet, wrist, ankle, and knee joints.

Diet has been strongly implicated in rheumatoid arthritis for many years, in regard to both cause and cure. The major focus in dietary therapy is to eliminate food allergies, follow a vegetarian diet, alter the intake of dietary fats and oils, and increase the intake of antioxidant nutrients. A long-term study conducted at the

Oslo Rheumatism Hospital showed that following these principles can be cura-
tive in some individuals with RA and significantly reduce symptoms in others.

The first step is a therapeutic fast or an elimination diet (see Food Allergy,
page 227), followed by careful reintroduction of foods to detect allergens.
Virtually any food can aggravate RA, but the most common offenders are
wheat, corn, milk and other dairy products, beef, and nightshade-family foods
(tomatoes, potatoes, eggplant, peppers, and tobacco). After isolating and eliminating all allergens, a healthy diet is recommended that is rich in whole foods,
vegetables, and fiber and low in sugar, meat, refined carbohydrates, and animal fats. Other important findings are:

- Eating cold-water fish, extra-virgin olive oil, and flavonoid-rich berries
  (cherries, hawthorn berries, blueberries, blackberries) helps alleviate RA.

- The importance of fresh fruits and vegetables in the dietary treatment
  of RA cannot be overstated. While the benefits of vitamin C, beta-
  carotene, vitamin E, selenium, and zinc as antioxidant nutrients are
  becoming well recognized and well accepted, there are still other plant
  compounds that promote healthy joints. Several studies have shown
  that the risk of RA is highest among people with the lowest levels of
  nutrient antioxidants (i.e., serum concentrations of vitamins C and E
  and beta-carotene).

- As stated elsewhere, vegetarian diets are often beneficial in the treatment
  of inflammatory conditions such as rheumatoid arthritis, presumably as
  a result of decreasing the availability of arachidonic acid for conversion
  to inflammatory compounds. Another important way of decreasing the
  inflammatory response is the consumption of cold-water fish. These
  fish are rich sources of long-chain omega-3 fatty acids. In addition, supplementing the diet with 1.8 to 3.0 grams of omega-3 fatty acids from a
  pharmaceutical-grade fish oil product is recommended.

- Fresh pineapple may provide some benefit due to the presence of bromelain, an anti-inflammatory enzyme. During flare-ups, fresh pineap-

ple juice and fresh ginger may help. Ginger exerts an anti-inflammatory action by inhibiting the manufacture of inflammatory compounds and by the presence of an anti-inflammatory enzyme similar to bromelain. In one clinical study, seven patients with rheumatoid arthritis in whom conventional drugs had provided only temporary or partial relief were treated with ginger. One patient took 50 grams per day of lightly cooked ginger, while the remaining six took either 5 grams of fresh or 0.1 to 1 gram of ground ginger daily. All patients reported substantial improvement, including pain relief, joint mobility, and decrease in swelling and morning stiffness.

Ulcer

An ulcer is a small wound that occurs in the stomach (gastric ulcer) or the first portion of the small intestine (duodenal ulcer).

Food allergy is a primary factor in many cases of peptic ulcer. A diet that eliminates food allergens has been used with great success in treating and preventing recurrent ulcers. It is especially important to avoid milk and dairy products. Milk is the most common food allergen, and population studies show that the higher the milk consumption, the greater the likelihood of developing an ulcer. Milk and coffee significantly increase stomach acid production; both should be avoided by individuals with ulcers. Other dietary factors include:

- A high-fiber diet is associated with a reduced rate of ulcers. Fiber supplements (pectin, guar gum, psyllium, etc.) have also been shown to produce beneficial effects.

- Raw cabbage juice is well documented as successful in treating peptic ulcers. In one study, drinking 1 liter of fresh cabbage juice throughout the day resulted in total ulcer healing in an average of ten days. The beneficial effect is thought to be due to the amino acid glutamine.

- Bananas, particularly plantains, may be of benefit due to their healing properties on the intestinal lining.

- Garlic, cayenne pepper, and turmeric may also be helpful due to their ability to inhibit the growth of the bacterium *Helicobacter pylori*, which is strongly linked to gastric ulcers.

Varicose Veins

Individuals with varicose veins have a decreased ability to break down fibrin. When fibrin is deposited in the tissue near the varicose veins, the skin becomes hard and "lumpy" due to the presence of the fibrin and fat. In addition, a decreased ability to break down fibrin increases the risk of thrombus formation, which may result in thrombophlebitis, heart attack, pulmonary embolism, or stroke. The most important dietary considerations are:

- A high-fiber diet is the most important component in the treatment and prevention of varicose veins (and hemorrhoids). A diet rich in vegetables, fruits, legumes, and grains promotes peristalsis; many fiber components attract water and form a gelatinous mass that keeps the feces soft, bulky, and easy to pass. Individuals who consume a low-fiber diet tend to strain more during bowel movements since their smaller and harder stools are more difficult to pass. This straining increases the pressure in the abdomen, which obstructs the flow of blood up the legs. The increased pressure may, over time, significantly weaken the walls of veins, leading to the formation of varicose veins.

- Flavonoid-rich berries, such as currants, blueberries, and blackberries, as well as cherries, are beneficial in the prevention and treatment of varicose veins. They are rich sources of flavonoids that improve the integrity of the support structures of the veins and entire vascular system.

Extracts of several of these berries are used widely in Europe as medications for various circulatory conditions, including varicose veins.

- Cayenne pepper, garlic, onions, and ginger all increase fibrin breakdown. Liberal consumption of these is recommended for individuals with varicose veins and other disorders of the cardiovascular system. In addition, bromelain, which is found in fresh pineapple, promotes the breakdown of fibrin.

Acknowledgments

Most important, I want to acknowledge all the researchers, physicians, and scientists who over the years have sought to better understand the magic of food and its impact on human health. Without their work, this book would certainly not exist. Next, I would like to acknowledge the support and efforts of everyone at Atria in putting this book together, led by Judith Curr. I greatly appreciate all of the hard work that went into the publication of this book. I would also like to express my gratitude to the DoctorMurray.com team, led by Michael Ebeling and Tabitha Moore, for their support. The same is also true for Scott Sensenbrenner and everyone else at Enzymedica. I am truly blessed to have such wonderful people to support my work whom I also can call my good friends. Thank you.

References

FOR THIRTY-SEVEN YEARS, I HAVE REVIEWED THOUSANDS OF SCIENTIFIC ARTICLES from medical journals on the healing power of foods and food components. The references provided do not represent a complete reference list of the studies mentioned in *The Magic of Food*. I have chosen to focus primarily on key studies and comprehensive review articles. I have also eliminated using the same reference twice. If you want more information or want to find out more details on the cited studies, access the Internet site of the National Library of Medicine (NLM), http://gateway.nlm.nih.gov.

At the NLM Gateway, users can search simultaneously in multiple retrieval systems. From this site you can access all of the NLM databases, including the PubMed database. This database was developed in conjunction with publishers of biomedical literature as a search tool for accessing literature citations and linking to full-text journal articles at web sites of participating publishers. Publishers participating in PubMed electronically supply NLM with their citations prior to or at the time of publication. If the publisher has a website that offers full text of its journals, PubMed provides links to that site, as well as sites to other biological data, sequence centers, etc. User registration, a subscription fee, or some other type of fee may be required to access the full text of articles in some journals.

PubMed provides access to bibliographic information that includes MEDLINE—the NLM's premier bibliographic database covering the fields of medicine, nursing, dentistry, veterinary medicine, the health care system, and the preclinical sciences. MEDLINE contains bibliographic citations and author abstracts from more than four thousand medical journals published in the United States and seventy other countries. The file contains more than fifteen million citations dating back to the mid-1960s. Coverage is worldwide, but most records are from English-language sources or have English abstracts (summaries). Conducting a search is quite easy, and the site has a link to a tutorial that fully explains the process.

1. You Are What You Eat

Nutrition and epigenetics:
Bishop K.S., Ferguson L.R. The interaction between epigenetics, nutrition and the development of cancer. *Nutrients*. (2015 Jan 30): 7(2): 922–47.
Pallauf K., Giller K., Huebbe P., Rimbach G. Nutrition and healthy ageing: calorie restriction or polyphenol-rich "MediterrAsian" diet? *Oxid Med Cell Longev*. (2013): 707421.
Remely M., Stefanska B., Lovrecic L., Magnet U., Haslberger A.G. Nu-triepigenomics: the role of nutrition in epigenetic control of human diseases. *Curr Opin Clin Nutr Metab Care*. (2015 Jul): 18(4): 328–33.
Smith C.J., Ryckman K.K. Epigenetic and developmental influences on the risk of obesity, diabetes, and metabolic syndrome. *Diabetes Metab Syndr Obes*. (2015 Jun 29): 8: 295–302.

2. What Should We Eat for Health and Longevity?

General references:
Cordain L., Eaton S.B., Miller J.B., et al. The paradoxical nature of hunter-gatherer diets: meat-based, yet non-atherogenic. *Eur J Clin Nutr*. (2002): 56(Suppl 1): S42–S52.
Eaton S.B., Eaton S.B. 3rd. Paleolithic vs. modern diets—selected patho-physiological implications. *Eur J Nutr*. (2000): 39: 67–70.

Katz D.L., Meller S. Can we say what diet is best for health? *Annu Rev Public Health.* (2014);35: 83–103.

Milton K. Nutritional characteristics of wild primate food: do the diets of our closest living relatives have lessons for us? *Nutrition.* (1999);15: 488–98.

Ryde D. What should humans eat? *Practitioner.* (1985): 232: 415–18.

Trowell H., Burkitt D. Western diseases: their emergence and prevention. Cambridge, MA: Harvard University Press, 1981.

The Seven Countries Study:

Menotti A., Puddu P.E. How the Seven Countries Study contributed to the definition and development of the Mediterranean diet concept: a 50-year journey. *Nutr Metab Cardiovasc Dis.* (2015 Mar): 25(3): 245–52.

Mediterranean diet protects against Alzheimer's disease and cognitive decline:

Feart C., Samieri C., Barberger-Gateau P. Mediterranean diet and cognitive health: an update of available knowledge. *Curr Opin Clin Nutr Metab Care.* (2015 Jan): 18(1): 51–62.

Safouris A., Tsivgoulis G., Sergentanis T.N., Psaltopoulou T. Mediterranean diet and risk of dementia. *Curr Alzheimer Res.* (2015): 12(8): 736–44.

The Okinawan diet:

Willcox D.C., Scapagnini G., Willcox B.J. Healthy aging diets other than the Mediterranean: a focus on the Okinawan diet. *Mech Ageing Dev.* (2014 Mar–Apr): 136–137: 148–62.

The New Nordic diet:

Fritzen A.M., Lundsgaard A.M., Jordy A.B. New Nordic diet induced weight loss is accompanied by changes in metabolism and AMPK signalling in adipose tissue. *J Clin Endocrinol Metab.* (2015 Jun 30): jc20152079.

Kolehmainen M., Ulven S.M., Paananen J., et al. Healthy Nordic diet downregulates the expression of genes involved in inflammation in subcutaneous adipose tissue in individuals with features of the metabolic syndrome. *Am J Clin Nutr.* (2015 Jan): 101(1): 228–39.

How diet affects epigenetic factors in Alzheimer's disease:

Dauncey M.J. Nutrition, the brain and cognitive decline: insights from epigenetics. *Eur J Clin Nutr.* (2014 Nov): 68(11): 1179–85.

Hanson A.J., Bayer-Carter J.L., Green P.S., et al. Effect of apolipoprotein E genotype and diet on apolipoprotein E lipidation and amyloid peptides: randomized clinical trial. *JAMA Neurol.* (2013 Jun 17): 1–9, doi:10.1001.

Lahiri D.K. Where the actions of environment (nutrition), gene and protein meet: beneficial role of fruit and vegetable juices in potentially delaying the onset of Alzheimer's disease. *J Alzheimers Dis.* (2006 Dec): 10(4): 359–61.

Phytochemicals that prevent Alzheimer's disease:

Bastianetto S., Krantic S., Quirion R. Polyphenols as potential inhibitors of amyloid aggregation and toxicity: possible significance to Alzheimer's disease. *Mini Rev Med Chem.* (2008 May): 8(5): 429–35.

Howes M.J., Perry E. The role of phytochemicals in the treatment and prevention of dementia. *Drugs Aging.* (2011 Jun 1): 28(6): 439–68.

Apples and Alzheimer's disease:

Chan A., Shea T.B. Dietary supplementation with apple juice decreases endogenous amyloid-beta levels in murine brain. *J Alzheimers Dis.* (2009): 16(1): 167–71.

Remington R., Chan A., Lepore A., Kotlya E., Shea T.B. Apple juice improved behavioral but not cognitive symptoms in moderate-to-late stage Alzheimer's disease in an open-label pilot study. *Am J Alzheimers Dis Other Demen.* (2010 Jun): 25(4): 367–71.

Dietary diversity and obesity risk:

Vadiveloo M., Dixon L.B., Mijanovich T., Elbel B., Parekh N. Dietary variety is inversely associated with body adiposity among US adults using a novel food diversity index. *J Nutr.* (2015 Mar): 145(3): 555–63.

3. AMPk: Activating the Enzyme of Youth, Longevity, and Weight Loss

Review articles on diet and AMPk:

Hwang J.T., Kwon D.Y., Yoon S.H. AMP-activated protein kinase: a potential target for the diseases prevention by natural occurring polyphenols. *N Biotechnol.* (2009 Oct 1): 26(1–2): 17–22.

McCarty M.F. AMPK activation—protean potential for boosting healthspan. *Age.* (Dordr). (2014 Apr): 36(2): 641–63.

Viollet B., Mounier R., Leclerc J., et al. Targeting AMP-activated protein kinase as a novel therapeutic approach for the treatment of metabolic disorders. *Diabetes Metab.* (2007 Dec): 33(6): 395–402.

Alpha-lipoic acid and weight loss:

Huerta A.E., Navas-Carretero S., Prieto-Hontoria P.L., Martínez J.A., Moreno-Aliaga M.J. Effects of a-lipoic acid and eicosapentaenoic acid in overweight and obese women during weight loss. *Obesity.* (2015 Feb): 23(2): 313–21.

Probiotics promote weight loss:

Sanchez M., Darimont C., Drapeau V., et al. Effect of Lactobacillus rhamnosus CGMCC1.3724 supplementation on weight loss and maintenance in obese men and women. *Br J Nutr.* (2014 Apr 28): 111(8): 1507–19.

Mediterranean diet and nut consumption:

Guasch-Ferré M., Bulló M., Martínez-González M.Á., et al. Frequency of nut consumption and mortality risk in the PREDIMED nutrition intervention trial. *BMC Med.* (2013 Jul 16): 11: 164.

Benefits of tagatose:

Espinosa I, Fogelfeld L. Tagatose: from a sweetener to a new diabetic medication? *Expert Opin Investig Drugs.* (2010 Feb): 19(2): 285–94.

4. Why Dietary Fats Are Essential

Avocado health benefits:

Dreher M.L., Davenport A.J. Hass avocado composition and potential health effects. *Crit Rev Food Sci Nutr.* (2013): 53(7): 738–50.

Fat and the human brain:

Bradbury J. Docosahexaenoic acid (DHA): an ancient nutrient for the modern human brain. *Nutrients.* (2011 May): 3(5): 529–54.

Brenna J.T., Carlson S.E. Docosahexaenoic acid and human brain development: evidence that a dietary supply is needed for optimal development. *J Hum Evol.* (2014 Dec): 77: 99–106, doi:10.1016/j.

Cunnane S.C., Crawford M.A. Energetic and nutritional constraints on infant brain development: implications for brain expansion during human evolution. *J Hum Evol.* (2014 Dec): 77: 88–98.

Pottala J.V., Yaffe K., Robinson J.G., et al. Higher RBC EPA + DHA corresponds with larger total brain and hippocampal volumes: WHIMS-MRI study. *Neurology.* (2014 Feb 4): 82(5): 435–42.

5. The Power of Plant Pigments

Vegetables and fruits contain the anticarcinogenic cocktail:

Steinmetz K.A., Potter J.D. Vegetables, fruits, and cancer. II. Mechanisms. *Cancer Causes Control.* (1991); 2: 427–42.

Health benefits of carotenes:

Gammone M.A., Riccioni G., D'Orazio N. Carotenoids: potential allies of cardiovascular health? *Food Nutr Res.* (2015 Feb 6); 59: 26762.

Krinsky N.I., Johnson E.J. Carotenoid actions and their relation to health and disease. *Mol Aspects Med.* (2005 Dec); 26(6): 459–516.

Astaxanthin the king of carotenes:

Ambati R.R., Phang S.M., Ravi S., Aswathanarayana R.G. Astaxanthin:

sources, extraction, stability, biological activities and its commercial applications—a review. *Mar Drugs.* (2014 Jan 7); 12(1): 128-52.

Fassett R.G., Coombes J.S. Astaxanthin in cardiovascular health and disease. *Molecules.* (2012 Feb 20); 17(2): 2030-48.

Kidd P. Astaxanthin, cell membrane nutrient with diverse clinical benefits and anti-aging potential. *Altern Med Rev.* (2011 Dec); 16(4): 355-64.

Flavonoids as nature's biological response modifiers:

Del Rio D., Rodriguez-Mateos A., Spencer J.P. Dietary (poly)phenolics in human health: structures, bioavailability, and evidence of protective effects against chronic diseases. *Antioxid Redox Signal.* (2013 May 10); 18(14): 1818 92.

Rodriguez-Mateos A., Vauzour D., Krueger C.G., Shanmuganayagam D., et al. Bioavailability, bioactivity and impact on health of dietary flavonoids and related compounds: an update. *Arch Toxicol.* (2014 Oct); 88(10): 1803-53.

Flavonoids and mortality:

Knekt P., Jarvinen R., Reunanen A., Maatela J. Flavonoid intake and coronary mortality in Finland: a cohort study. *BMJ.* (1996); 312 (7029): 478-81.

Macready A.L., George T.W., Chong M.F., et al. Flavonoid-rich fruits and vegetables improve microvascular reactivity and inflammatory status in men at risk of cardiovascular disease—FLAVURS: a randomized controlled trial. *Am J Clin Nutr.* (2014 Mar); 99(3): 479-89.

McCullough M.L., Peterson J.J., Patel R., Flavonoid intake and cardiovascular disease mortality in a prospective cohort of US adults. *Am J Clin Nutr.* (2012 Feb); 95(2): 454-64.

Fruit intake protects against diabetes:

Muraki I., Imamura F., Manson J.E., et al. Fruit consumption and risk of type 2 diabetes: results from three prospective longitudinal cohort studies. *BMJ.* (2013 Aug 28); 347: f5001. doi:10.1136/bmj.f5001.

Boron reduces calcium excretion:

Neilsen F.H., Hunt C.D., Mullen L.M., Hunt J.R. Effect of dietary boron on mineral, estrogen, and testosterone metabolism in postmenopausal women. *FASEB J.* (1987); 1: 394–7.

Spinach protects against breast cancer:

Longnecker M.P., Newcomb P.A., Mittendorf R., et al. Intake of carrots, spinach, and supplements containing vitamin A in relation to risk of breast cancer. *Cancer Epidemiol Biomarkers Prev.* (1997); 6(11): 887–92.

Mangoes' health benefits:

Drammeh B.S., Marquis G.S., Funkhouser E., Bates C., Eto I., Stephensen C.B. A randomized, 4-month mango and fat supplementation trial improved vitamin A status among young Gambian children. *J Nutr.* (2002); 132(12): 3693–9.

Pandey M., Shukla V.K. Diet and gallbladder cancer: a case-control study. *Eur J Cancer Prev.* (2002 Aug); 11(4): 365–8.

Percival S.S., Talcott S.T., Chin S.T., et al. Neoplastic transformation of BALB/3T3 cells and cell cycle of HL-60 cells are inhibited by mango (Mangifera indica L.) juice and mango juice extracts. *J Nutr.* (2006 May); 136(5): 1300–4.

Lemons fight cancer:

Crowell P.L. Prevention and therapy of cancer by dietary monoterpenes. *J Nutr.* (1999 Mar); 129(3): 775S–778S.

Miller J.A., Lang J.E., Ley M., et al. Human breast tissue disposition and bioactivity of limonene in women with early stage breast cancer. *Cancer Prev Res* (Phila). (2013 Jun); 6(6): 577–84.

Beet juice lowers blood pressure:

Asgary S., Afshani M.R., Sahebkar A., et al. Improvement of hypertension, endothelial function and systemic inflammation following short-term supplementation with red beet (Beta vulgaris L.) juice: a randomized crossover pilot study. *J Hum Hypertens*. (2016 Jun 9). doi:10.1038/jhh.2016.34.

Coles L.T., Clifton P.M. Effect of beetroot juice on lowering blood pressure in free-living, disease-free adults: a randomized, placebo-controlled trial. *Nutrition Journal*. (2012); 11:106 doi:10.1186/1475-2891-11-106.

Siervo M., Lara J., Ogbonmwan I., Mathers J.C. Inorganic nitrate and beetroot juice supplementation reduces blood pressure in adults: a systematic review and meta-analysis. *J Nutr*. (2013 Jun); 143(6): 818–26.

Blueberries' health benefits:

Cassidy A., Mukamal K.J., Liu L., et al. High anthocyanin intake is associated with a reduced risk of myocardial infarction in young and middle-aged women. *Circulation*. (2013 Jan 15); 127(2): 188–96.

Giacalone M., Di Sacco F., Traupe I., et al. Antioxidant and neuroprotective properties of blueberry polyphenols: a critical review. *Nutr Neurosci*. (2011 May); 14(3): 119–25.

Johnson S.A., Arjmandi B.H. Evidence for anti-cancer properties of blueberries: a mini-review. *Anticancer Agents Med Chem*. (2013 Oct); 13(8): 1142–8.

Cherries fight gout:

Jacob R.A., Spinozzi G.M., Simon V.A., et al. Consumption of cherries lowers plasma urate in healthy women. *J Nutr*. (2003); 133(6): 1826–9.

Kelley D.S., Rasooly R., Jacob R.A., Kader A.A., Mackey B.E. Consumption of Bing sweet cherries lowers circulating concentrations of inflammation markers in healthy men and women. *J Nutr*. (2006 Apr); 136(4): 981–6.

Zhang Y., Neogi T., Chen C., et al. Cherry consumption and the risk of recurrent gout attacks. *Arthritis Rheum*. (2012 Sep 28). doi:10.1002/art.346718.

Strawberries and cholesterol:

Basu A., Betts N.M., Nguyen A., et al. Freeze-dried strawberries lower serum cholesterol and lipid peroxidation in adults with abdominal adiposity and elevated serum lipids. *J Nutr*. (2014 Jun); 144(6): 830–7.

Lycopene's health benefits:

Chen J., Song Y., Zhang L. Effect of lycopene supplementation on oxidative stress: an exploratory systematic review and meta-analysis of randomized controlled trials. *J Med Food.* (2013 May); 16(5): 361–74.

Giovannucci E., Rimm E.B., Liu Y., Stampfer M.J., Willett W.C. A prospective study of tomato products, lycopene, and prostate cancer risk. *J Natl Cancer Inst.* (2002); 94(5): 391–8.

Perveen R., Suleria H.A., Anjum F.M., et al. Tomato (*Solanum lycopersicum*) carotenoids and lycopenes chemistry; metabolism, absorption, nutrition, and allied health claims—a comprehensive review. *Crit Rev Food Sci Nutr.* (2015); 55(7): 919–29.

Rao A.V., Agarwal S. Role of antioxidant lycopene in cancer and heart disease. *J Am Coll Nutr.* (2000); 19(5): 563–9.

Weisburger J.H. Lycopene and tomato products in health promotion. *Exp Biol Med.* (2002); 227(10): 924–7.

Watermelon juice relieves muscle soreness:

Tarazona-Díaz M.P., Alacid F., Carrasco M., Martínez I., Aguayo E. Watermelon juice: potential functional drink for sore muscle relief in athletes. *J Agric Food Chem.* (2013 Aug 7); 61(31): 7522–8.

6. My Favorite Superfoods

Green tea and cancer:

Butt M.S., Ahmad R.S., Sultan M.T., Qayyum M.M., Naz A. Green tea and anticancer perspectives: updates from last decade. *Crit Rev Food Sci Nutr.* (2015); 55(6): 792–805.

Lambert J.D. Does tea prevent cancer? Evidence from laboratory and human intervention studies. *Am J Clin Nutr.* (2013 Dec); 98(6 Suppl): 1667S–1675S.

Ogunleye A.A., Xue F., Michels K.B. Green tea consumption and breast cancer risk or recurrence: a meta-analysis. *Breast Cancer Res Treat.* (2010); 119: 477–84.

Berries:

Afrin S., Giampieri F., Gasparrini M. et al. Chemopreventive and therapeutic effects of edible berries: a focus on colon cancer prevention and treatment. *Molecules.* (2016 Jan 30); 21(2): 169.

Cerletti C., de Curtis A., Bracone F. et al. Dietary anthocyanins and health: data from FLORA and ATHENA EU projects. *Br J Clin Pharmacol.* (2016 Mar 25). doi:10.1111/bcp.12943.

Del Bo' C., Martini D., Porrini M., Klimis-Zacas D., Riso P. Berries and oxidative stress markers: an overview of human intervention studies. *Food Funct.* (2015 Sep); 6(9): 2890–917.

Del Rio D., Borges G., Crozier A. Berry flavonoids and phenolics: bioavailability and evidence of protective effects. *Br J Nutr.* (2010 Oct); 104 Suppl 3: S67–90.

Lasekan O. Exotic berries as a functional food. *Curr Opin Clin Nutr Metab Care.* (2014 Nov); 17(6): 589–95.

Rodriguez-Mateos A., Heiss C., Borges G., Crozier A. Berry (poly)phenols and cardiovascular health. *J Agric Food Chem.* (2014 May 7); 62(18): 3842–51.

Skrovankova S., Sumczynski D., Mlcek J., Jurikova T., Sochor J. Bioactive compounds and antioxidant activity in different types of berries. *Int J Mol Sci.* (2015 Oct 16);16(10): 24673–706.

Tsuda T. Recent progress in anti-obesity and anti-diabetes effect of berries. *Antioxidants* (Basel). (2016 Apr 6); 5(2). pii: E13.

Variya B.C., Bakrania A.K., Patel S.S. Emblica officinalis (Amla): a review for its phytochemistry, ethnomedicinal uses and medicinal potentials with respect to molecular mechanisms. *Pharmacol Res.* (2016 Jun 15); 111: 180–200.

Zia-Ul-Haq M., Riaz M., De Feo V., Jaafar H.Z., Moga M. Rubus fruticosus L.: constituents, biological activities and health related uses. *Molecules.* (2014 Jul 28); 19(8): 10998–1029.

Black currants:

Gopalan A., Reuben S.C., Ahmed S., et al. The health benefits of blackcurrants. *Food Funct.* (2012 Aug); 3(8): 795–809.

Cranberries:

Blumberg J.B., Camesano T.A., Cassidy A., et al. Cranberries and their bioactive constituents in human health. *Adv Nutr.* (2013 Nov 6); 4(6): 618–32.

Zhu Y., Miao Y., Meng Z., Zhong Y. Effects of vaccinium berries on serum lipids: a meta-analysis of randomized controlled trials. *Evid Based Complement Alternat Med.* (2015): 790329.

Raspberries:

Burton-Freeman B.M., Sandhu A.K., Edirisinghe I. Red raspberries and their bioactive polyphenols: cardiometabolic and neuronal health links. *Adv Nutr.* (2016 Jan 15); 7(1): 44–65.

Strawberries:

Afrin S., Gasparrini M., Forbes-Hernandez T.Y., Reboredo-Rodriguez P., et al. Promising health benefits of the strawberry: a focus on clinical studies. *J Agric Food Chem.* (2016 Jun 8); 64(22): 4435–49.

Giampieri F., Forbes-Hernandez T.Y., Gasparrini M., et al. Strawberry as a health promoter: an evidence based review. *Food Funct.* (2015 May); 6(5): 1386–98.

Hannum S.M. Potential impact of strawberries on human health: a review of the science. *Crit Rev Food Sci Nutr.* (2004); 44(1): 1–17.

Grapes:

Nassiri-Asl M., Hosseinzadeh H. Review of the pharmacological effects of Vitis vinifera (grape) and its bioactive constituents: an update. *Phytother Res.* (2016 May 16). doi:10.1002/ptr.5644.

Wightman J.D., Heuberger R.A. Effect of grape and other berries on cardiovascular health. *J Sci Food Agric.* (2015 Jun); 95(8): 1584–97.

Pomegranate:

Aviram M., Rosenblat M., Gaitini D., et al. Pomegranate juice consumption for 3 years by patients with carotid artery stenosis reduces common carotid intima-media thickness, blood pressure and LDL oxidation. *Clin Nutr.* (2004); 23(3): 423–33.

Medjakovic S., Jungbauer A. Pomegranate: a fruit that ameliorates metabolic syndrome. *Food Funct.* (2013 Jan); 4(1): 19–39.

Sumner M.D., Elliott-Eller M., Weidner G., et al. Effects of pomegranate juice consumption on myocardial perfusion in patients with coronary heart disease. *Am J Cardiol.* (2005); 96(6): 810–14.

Syed D.N., Chamcheu J.C., Adhami V.M., Mukhtar H. Pomegranate extracts and cancer prevention: molecular and cellular activities. *Anticancer Agents Med Chem.* (2013 Oct); 13(8): 1149–61. Review.

Zarfeshany A., Asgary S., Javanmard S.H. Potent health effects of pomegranate. *Adv Biomed Res.* (2014 Mar 25); 3: 100.

Raw cacao powder and dark chocolate:

Cocoa flavonols' and dark chocolate's general health benefits:

Ellam S., Williamson G. Cocoa and human health. *Annu Rev Nutr.* (2013); 33: 105–28.

Ellinger S., Stehle P. Impact of cocoa consumption on inflammation processes—a critical review of randomized controlled trials. *Nutrients.* (2016 May 26); 8(6). pii: E321.

Goya L., Martín M.Á., Sarriá B., Ramos S., Mateos R., Bravo L. Effect of cocoa and its flavonoids on biomarkers of inflammation: studies of cell culture, animals and humans. *Nutrients.* (2016 Apr 9); 8(4).

Hooper L., Kay C., Abdelhamid A. et al. Effects of chocolate, cocoa, and flavan-3-ols on cardiovascular health: a systematic review and meta-analysis of randomized trials. *Am J Clin Nutr.* (2012 Mar); 95(3): 740–51.

Kim J., Kim J., Shim J. et al. Cocoa phytochemicals: recent advances in molecular mechanisms on health. *Crit Rev Food Sci Nutr.* (2014); 54(11): 1458–72.

Latham L.S., Hensen Z.K., Minor D.S. Chocolate—guilty pleasure or healthy supplement? *J Clin Hypertens* (Greenwich). (2014 Feb); 16(2): 101–6. Review.

Latif R. Health benefits of cocoa. *Curr Opin Clin Nutr Metab Care.* (2013 Nov); 16(6): 669–74. doi:10.

Cocoa flavonols and dark chocolate improve brain function:

Lamport D.J., Pal D., Moutsiana C., Field D.T., et al. The effect of flava-
nol-rich cocoa on cerebral perfusion in healthy older adults during con-
scious resting state: a placebo controlled, crossover, acute trial. *Psycho-
pharmacology* (Berl). (2015 Sep); 232(17): 3227–34.

Scholey A., Owen L. Effects of chocolate on cognitive function and mood: a
systematic review. *Nutr Rev.* (2013 Oct); 71(10): 665–81.

Sokolov A.N., Pavlova M.A., Klosterhalfen S., Enck P. Chocolate and the
brain: neurobiological impact of cocoa flavanols on cognition and behavior. *Neurosci Biobehav Rev.* (2013 Dec); 37(10 Pt 2): 2445–53.

Sorond F.A., Hurwitz S., Salat D.H., Greve D.N., Fisher N.D. Neurovascular coupling, cerebral white matter integrity, and response to cocoa in
older people. *Neurology.* (2013 Sep 3); 81(10): 904–9.

Green tea:

Afzal M., Safer A.M., Menon M. Green tea polyphenols and their potential
role in health and disease. *Inflammopharmacology.* (2015 Aug); 23(4):
151–61.

Khan N., Mukhtar H. Tea and health: studies in humans. *Curr Pharm Des.*
(2013);19(34): 6141–7.

Tenore G.C., Daglia M., Ciampaglia R., Novellino E. Exploring the nutra-
ceutical potential of polyphenols from black, green and white tea infu-
sions—an overview. *Curr Pharm Biotechnol.* (2015); 16(3): 265–71.

Green tea and prostate cancer:

Bettuzzi S., Brausi M., Rizzi F., et al. Chemoprevention of human prostate
cancer by oral administration of green tea catechins in volunteers with
high-grade prostate intraepithelial neoplasia: a preliminary report from a
one-year proof-of-principle study. *Cancer Res.* (2006); 66: 1234–40.

Thomas R., Williams M., Sharma H., Chaudry A., Bellamy P. A double-blind, placebo-controlled randomised trial evaluating the effect of
a polyphenol-rich whole food supplement on PSA progression in men
with prostate cancer—the U.K. NCRN Pomi-T study. *Prostate Cancer
Prostatic Dis.* (2014 Jun); 17(2): 180–6.

McLarty J., Bigelow R.L., Smith M., et al. Tea polyphenols decrease serum levels of prostate-specific antigen, hepatocyte growth factor, and vascular endothelial growth factor in prostate cancer patients and inhibit production of hepatocyte growth factor and vascular endothelial growth factor in vitro. *Cancer Prev Res* (Phila). (2009); 2: 673–82.

Wang P., Aronson W.J., Huang M., et al. Green tea polyphenols and metabolites in prostatectomy tissue: implications for cancer prevention. *Cancer Prev Res* (Phila). (2010); 3: 985–93.

L-theanine:

Cooper R. Green tea and theanine: health benefits. *Int J Food Sci Nutr.* (2012 Mar); 63 Suppl 1: 90–7.

Nathan P.J., Lu K., Gray M., Oliver C. The neuropharmacology of L-theanine (N-ethyl-L-glutamine): a possible neuroprotective and cognitive enhancing agent. *J Herb Pharmacother.* (2006); 6: 21–30.

Bee pollen:

Komosinska-Vassev K., Olczyk P., Każmierczak J., Mencner L., Olczyk K. Bee pollen: chemical composition and therapeutic application. *Evid Based Complement Alternat Med.* (2015); 2015: 297425.

Rzepecka-Stojko A., Stojko J., Kurek-Górecka A., et al. Polyphenols from bee pollen: structure, absorption, metabolism and biological activity. *Molecules.* (2015 Dec 4); 20(12): 21732–49.

Ground flaxseed:

Demark-Wahnefried W., Polascik T.J., George S.L. et al. Flaxseed supplementation (not dietary fat restriction) reduces prostate cancer proliferation rates in men presurgery. *Cancer Epidemiol Biomarkers Prev.* (2008 Dec); 17(12): 3577–87.

Edel A.L., Rodriguez-Leyva D., Maddaford T.G., et al. Dietary flaxseed independently lowers circulating cholesterol and lowers it beyond the effects of cholesterol-lowering medications alone in patients with peripheral artery disease. *J Nutr.* (2015 Apr); 145(4): 749–57.

Goyal A., Sharma V., Upadhyay N., Gill S., Sihag M. Flax and flaxseed oil: an ancient medicine & modern functional food. *J Food Sci Technol.* (2014 Sep); 51(9): 1633–53.

Kajla P., Sharma A., Sood D.R. Flaxseed—a potential functional food source. *J Food Sci Technol.* (2015 Apr); 52(4): 1857–71.

Maddaford T.G., Ramjiawan B., Aliani M., Guzman R., Pierce G.N. Potent antihypertensive action of dietary flaxseed in hypertensive patients. *Hypertension.* (2013 Dec); 62(6): 1081–9.

Mason J.K., Thompson L.U. Flaxseed and its lignan and oil components: can they play a role in reducing the risk of and improving the treatment of breast cancer? *Appl Physiol Nutr Metab.* (2014 Jun); 39(6): 663–78.

Whey protein:

Akhavan T., Luhovyy B.L., Panahi S., et al. Mechanism of action of pre-meal consumption of whey protein on glycemic control in young adults. *J Nutr Biochem.* (2014 Jan); 25(1): 36–43.

Baer D.J., Stote K.S., Paul D.R., et al. Whey protein but not soy protein supplementation alters body weight and composition in free-living overweight and obese adults. *J Nutr.* (2011); 141(8): 1489–94.

Hector A.J., Marcotte G.R., Churchward-Venne T.A., et al. Whey protein supplementation preserves postprandial myofibrillar protein synthesis during short-term energy restriction in overweight and obese adults. *J Nutr.* (2015 Feb); 145(2): 246–52.

PolyGlycopleX (PGX):

Brand-Miller J.C., Atkinson F.S., Gahler R.J., et al. Effects of PGX, a novel functional fibre, on acute and delayed postprandial glycaemia. *Eur J Clin Nutr.* (2010 Dec); 64(12): 1488–93.

Jenkins A.L., Kacinik V., Lyon M.R., Wolever T.M.S. Reduction of postprandial glycemia by the novel viscous polysaccharide PGX in a dose-dependent manner, independent of food form. *J Am Coll Nutr.* (2010); 29(2): 92–8.

Lyon M.R., Reichert R.G. The effect of a novel viscous polysaccharide along with lifestyle changes on short-term weight loss and associated risk factors in overweight and obese adults: an observational retrospective clinical program analysis. *Altern Med Rev.* (2010 Apr); 15(1): 68–75.

Reimer R.A., Pelletier X., Carabin I.G., et al. Increased plasma PYY levels following supplementation with the functional fiber PolyGlycopleX in healthy adults. *Eur J Clin Nutr.* (2010 Oct); 64(10): 1186–91.

Solah V.A., Brand-Miller J.C., Atkinson F.S., et al. Dose-response effect of a novel functional fibre, PolyGlycopleX®, PGX®, on satiety. *Appetite.* (2014 Mar 12); doi:10.1016/j.appet.2014.02.021.

Vuksan V., Sievenpiper J.L., Owen R., et al. Beneficial effects of viscous dietary fiber from Konjac-mannan in subjects with the insulin resistance syndrome: results of a controlled metabolic trial. *Diabetes Care.* (2000); 23: 9–14.

Yong M.K., Solah V.A., Johnson S.K., et al. Effects of a viscous-fibre supplemented evening meal and the following un-supplemented breakfast on post-prandial satiety responses in healthy women, *Physiology & Behavior.* (2015); doi:10.1016/j.physbeh.2015.11.006.

7. Spice It Up!

General:

Howes M.J., Simmonds M.S. The role of phytochemicals as micronutrients in health and disease. *Curr Opin Clin Nutr Metab Care.* (2014 Nov); 17(6): 558–6.

Saldanha L.G., Dwyer J.T., Betz J.M. Culinary spice plants in dietary supplement products and tested in clinical trials. *Adv Nutr.* (2016 Mar 15); 7(2): 343–8.

Black pepper:

Meghwal M., Goswami T.K. Piper nigrum and piperine: an update. *Phytother Res.* (2013 Aug); 27(8): 1121–30.

Srinivasan K. Black pepper and its pungent principle-piperine: a review of diverse physiological effects. *Crit Rev Food Sci Nutr.* (2007); 47(8): 735–48.

Cayenne pepper:

Ahuja K.D., Robertson I.K., Geraghty D.P., Ball M.J. The effect of 4-week chili supplementation on metabolic and arterial function in humans. *Eur J Clin Nutr*. (2007 Mar); 61(3): 326–33.

Ahuja K.D., Robertson I.K., Geraghty D.P., Ball M.J. Effects of chili consumption on postprandial glucose, insulin, and energy metabolism. *Am J Clin Nutr*. (2006 Jul); 84(1): 63–9.

Bortolotti M., Coccia G., Grossi G. Red pepper and functional dyspepsia. *New Engl J Med*. (2002); 346: 947–8.

Bortolotti M., Porta S. Effect of red pepper on symptoms of irritable bowel syndrome: preliminary study. *Dig Dis Sci*. (2011 Nov); 56(11): 3288–95.

Gonzalez R., Dunkel R., Koletzko B., et al. Effect of capsaicin-containing red pepper sauce suspension on upper gastrointestinal motility in healthy volunteers. *Dig Dis Sci*. (1998); 43(6): 1165–71.

Khan F.A., Mahmood T., Ali M., Saeed A., Maalik A. Pharmacological importance of an ethnobotanical plant: Capsicum annuum L. *Nat Prod Res*. (2014); 28(16): 1267–74.

Nieman D.C., Cialdella-Kam L., Knab A.M., Shanely R.A. Influence of red pepper spice and turmeric on inflammation and oxidative stress biomarkers in overweight females: a metabolomics approach. *Plant Foods Hum Nutr*. (2012 Dec); 67(4): 415–21.

Rodriguez-Stanley S., Collings K.L., Robinson M., Owen W., Miner P.B. Jr. The effects of capsaicin on reflux, gastric emptying and dyspepsia. *Aliment Pharmacol Ther*. (2000); 14(1): 129–34.

Sambaiah K., Satyanarayana M.N. Hypocholesterolemic effect of red pepper & capsaicin. *Indian J Exp Biol*. (1980); 18(8): 898–9.

Visudhiphan S., Poolsuppasit S., Piboonnakarintr O., Tumliang S. The relationship between high fibrinolytic activity and daily capsicum ingestion in Thais. *Am J Clin Nutr*. (1982); 35: 1452–8.

Mustard:

Fujioka N., Fritz V., Upadhyaya P., Kassie F., Hecht S.S. Research on cruciferous vegetables, indole-3-carbinol, and cancer prevention: a tribute to

Lee W. Wattenberg. *Mol Nutr Food Res.* (2016 Jun); 60(6): 1228–38.

Gupta P., Wright S.E., Kim S.H., Srivastava S.K. Phenethyl isothiocyanate: a comprehensive review of anti-cancer mechanisms. *Biochim Biophys Acta.* (2014 Dec); 1846(2): 405–24.

Kumar G., Tuli H.S., Mittal S., et al. Isothiocyanates: a class of bioactive metabolites with chemopreventive potential. *Tumour Biol.* (2015 Jun); 36(6): 4005–16.

Mazumder A., Dwivedi A., du Plessis J. Sinigrin and its therapeutic benefits. *Molecules.* (2016 Mar 29); 21(4). pii: E416.

Turmeric:

Aggarwal B.B., Yuan W., Li S., Gupta S.C. Curcumin-free turmeric exhibits anti-inflammatory and anticancer activities: identification of novel components of turmeric. *Mol Nutr Food Res.* (2013 Sep); 57(9): 1529–42.

Ghosh S., Banerjee S., Sil P.C. The beneficial role of curcumin on inflammation, diabetes and neurodegenerative disease: a recent update. *Food Chem Toxicol.* (2015 Sep); 83: 111–24.

Gupta S.C., Sung B., Kim J.H., Prasad S., Li S., Aggarwal B.B. Multitargeting by turmeric, the golden spice: from kitchen to clinic. *Mol Nutr Food Res.* (2013 Sep); 57(9): 1510–28.

Jeenger M.K., Shrivastava S., Yerra V.G., et al. Curcumin: a pleiotropic phytonutrient in diabetic complications. *Nutrition.* (2015 Feb); 31(2): 276–82.

Shanmugam M.K., Rane G., Kanchi M.M., et al. The multifaceted role of curcumin in cancer prevention and treatment. *Molecules.* (2015 Feb 5); 20(2): 2728–69.

Shimouchi A., Nose K., Takaoka M., Hayashi H., Kondo T. Effect of dietary turmeric on breath hydrogen. *Dig Dis Sci.* (2009 Aug); 54(8): 1725–9.

Trujillo J., Granados-Castro L.F., Zazueta C. Mitochondria as a target in the therapeutic properties of curcumin. *Arch Pharm* (Weinheim). (2014 Dec); 347(12): 873–84.

Mint:

Elgayyar M., Draughon F.A., Golden D.A., Mount J.R. Antimicrobial activity of essential oils from plants against selected pathogenic and saprophytic microorganisms. *J Food Prot.* (2001); 64(7): 1019–24.

Keifer D., Ulbricht C., Abrams T.R., et al. Peppermint (Mentha piperita): an evidence-based systematic review by the Natural Standard Research Collaboration. *J Herb Pharmacother.* (2007); 7(2): 91–143.

Lagouri V., Boskou D. Nutrient antioxidants in oregano. *Int J Food Sci Nutr.* (1996); 47(6): 493–7.

Martinez-Tome M., Jimenez A.M., Ruggieri S., Frega N., Strabbioli R., Murcia M.A. Antioxidant properties of Mediterranean spices compared with common food additives. *J Food Prot.* (2001); 64(9): 1412–19.

Zheng W., Wang S.Y. Antioxidant activity and phenolic compounds in selected herbs. *J Agric Food Chem.* (2001); 49(11): 5165–70.

Sodium and potassium:

Khaw K.T., Barrett-Connor E. Dietary potassium and stroke-associated mortality. *N Engl J Med.* (1987); 316: 235–40.

Jansson B. Dietary, total body, and intracellular potassium-to-sodium ratios and their influence on cancer. *Cancer Detect Prevent.* (1991); 14: 563–5.

Whelton P.K., He J. Potassium in preventing and treating high blood pressure. *Semin Nephrol.* (1999); 19: 494–9.

Garlic:

Nicastro H.L., Ross S.A., Milner J.A. Garlic and onions: their cancer prevention properties. *Cancer Prev Res* (Phila). (2015 Mar); 8(3): 181–9.

Rana S.V., Pal R., Vaiphei K., Sharma S.K., Ola R.P. Garlic in health and disease. *Nutr Res.* (Rev. 2011 Jun); 24(1): 60–71.

Ried K. Garlic lowers blood pressure in hypertensive individuals, regulates serum cholesterol, and stimulates immunity: an updated meta-analysis and review. *J Nutr.* (2016 Feb); 146(2): 389S–396S.

Sainani G.S., Desai D.B., Gohre N.H., et al. Effect of dietary garlic and onion on serum lipid profile in Jain community. *Ind J Med Res.* (1979); 69: 776–80.

Varshney R., Budoff M.J. Garlic and heart disease. *J Nutr.* (2016 Feb); 146(2): 416S–421S.

Xiong X.J., Wang P.Q., Li S.J., et al. Garlic for hypertension: a systematic review and meta-analysis of randomized controlled trials. *Phytomedicine.* (2015 Mar 15); 22(3): 352–61.

Ginger:

Al-Nahain A., Jahan R., Rahmatullah M. *Zingiber officinale:* a potential plant against rheumatoid arthritis. *Arthritis.* 2014: 159089.

Kubra I.R., Rao L.J. An impression on current developments in the technology, chemistry, and biological activities of ginger (Zingiber officinale Roscoe). *Crit Rev Food Sci Nutr.* (2012); 52(8): 651–88.

Lakhan S.E., Ford C.T., Tepper D. Zingiberaceae extracts for pain: a systematic review and meta-analysis. *Nutr J.* (2015 May 14); 14: 50.

Lete I., Allué J. The effectiveness of ginger in the prevention of nausea and vomiting during pregnancy and chemotherapy. *Integr Med Insights.* (2016 Mar 31); 11: 11–17.

Maghbooli M., Golipour F., Moghimi Esfandabadi A., Yousefi M. Comparison between the efficacy of ginger and sumatriptan in the ablative treatment of the common migraine. *Phytother Res.* (2014 Mar); 28(3): 412–15.

Viljoen E., Visser J., Koen N., Musekiwa A. A systematic review and meta-analysis of the effect and safety of ginger in the treatment of pregnancy-associated nausea and vomiting. *Nutr J.* (2014 Mar 19); 13: 20.

Sugar:

Lennerz B.S., Alsop D.C., Holsen L.M., et al. Effects of dietary glycemic index on brain regions related to reward and craving in men. *Am J Clin Nutr.* (2013 Jun 26). doi:10.3945.

8. The Synergetic Diet with Recipes

Hollis J.F., Gullion C.M., Stevens V.J., et al. Importance of menu planning and a food diary: weight loss during the intensive intervention phase of the weight-loss maintenance trial. *Am J Prev Med.* (2008 Aug); 35(2): 118–26.

Fresh juice versus pasteurized juice:

Bakkalbasi E., Mentes O., Artik N. Food ellagitannins—occurrence, effects of processing and storage. *Crit Rev Food Sci Nutr.* (2009 Mar); 49(3): 283–98.

Gerhauser C. Cancer chemopreventive potential of apples, apple juice, and apple components. *Planta Med.* (2008); 74: 1608–24.

Konowalchuk J., Speirs J.I. Antiviral effect of apple beverages. *Appl Envir Microbiol.* (1978); 36: 798–801.

Soler C., Soriano J.M., Mañes J. Apple-products phytochemicals and processing: a review. *Nat Prod Commun.* (2009 May); 4(5): 659–70.

9. Food as Medicine

Acne:

Berra B., Rizzo A.M. Glycemic index, glycemic load: new evidence for a link with acne. *J Am Coll Nutr.* (2009 Aug); 28 Suppl: 450S–454S.

Cordain L., Lindeberg S., Hurtado M., et al. Acne vulgaris: a disease of Western civilization. *Arch Dermatol.* (2002); 138: 1584–90.

Danby F.W. Nutrition and acne. *Clin Dermatol.* (2010 Nov–Dec); 28(6): 598–604.

Grover R.W., Arikan N. The effect of intralesional insulin and glucagon in acne vulgaris. *L Invest Derm.* (1963); 40: 259–61.

Kader M.M., El-Mofty A.M., Ismail A.A,. Bassili F. Glucose tolerance in blood and skin of patients with acne vulgaris. *Ind J Derm.* (1977); 22: 139–49.

Melnik B.C., Schmitz G. Role of insulin, insulin-like growth factor-1, hyperglycaemic food and milk consumption in the pathogenesis of acne vulgaris. *Exp Dermatol.* (2009 Oct); 18(10): 833–41.

Seleit I., Bakry O.A., Abdou A.G., Hashim A. Body mass index, selected dietary factors, and acne severity: are they related to in situ expression of insulin-like growth factor-1? *Anal Quant Cytopathol Histpathol.* (2014 Oct); 36(5): 267–78.

Semon H., Herrmann F. Some observations on the sugar metabolism in acne vulgaris, and its treatment by insulin. *Br J Derm.* (1940); 52: 123–8.

Alzheimer's disease:

Morris M.C., Tangney C.C., Wang Y., et al. MIND diet slows cognitive decline with aging. *Alzheimers Dement.* (2015 Sep); 11(9): 1015–22.

Anxiety:

Bruce M., Lader M. Caffeine abstention in the management of anxiety disorders. *Psychol Med.* (1989); 19: 211–14.

Charney D., Heninger G., Jatlow P. Increased anxiogenic effects of caffeine in panic disorders. *Arch Gen Psychiatry.* (1985); 42: 233–43.

Green P., Hermesh H., Monselise A., et al. Red cell membrane omega-3 fatty acids are decreased in nondepressed patients with social anxiety disorder. *Eur Neuropsychopharmacol.* (2006); 16: 107–13.

Kiecolt-Glasera J.K., Beluryc M.A., Andridged R., Malarkeya W.B., Glasera R. Omega-3 supplementation lowers inflammation and anxiety in medical students: a randomized controlled trial. *Brain Behavior Immunity.* (July 2011). doi:10.1016/j.bbi.2011.07.229.

Asthma:

Britton J., Pavord I., Richards K., et al. Dietary magnesium, lung function, wheezing, and airway hyper-reactivity in a random adult population sample. *Lancet.* (1994); 344: 357–62.

Businco L., Falconieri P., Giampietro P., et al. Food allergy and asthma. *Pediatr Pulmonol Suppl.* (1995); 11: 59–60.

Carrey O.J., Locke C., Cookson J.B. Effect of alterations of dietary sodium on the severity of asthma in men. *Thorax.* (1993); 48: 714–18.

Denny S.I., Thompson R.L., Margetts B.M. Dietary factors in the pathogenesis of asthma and chronic obstructive pulmonary disease. *Curr Allergy Asthma Rep.* (2003); 3: 130–6.

Dry J., Vincent D. Effect of a fish oil diet on asthma. Results of a 1-year double-blind study. *Int Arch Allergy Apply Immunol.* (1991); 95: 156–57.

Freedman B.J. A diet free from additives in the management of allergic disease. *Clin Allergy.* (1977); 7: 417–21.

Hodge L., Salome C.M., Peat J.K., et al. Consumption of oily fish and childhood asthma risk. *Med J Aust.* (1996); 164: 137–40.

Lau B.H., Riesen S.K., Truong K.P., et al. Pycnogenol as an adjunct in the management of childhood asthma. *J Asthma.* (2004); 41(8): 825–32.

Lindahl O., Lindwall L., Spangberg A., et al. Vegan diet regimen with reduced medication in the treatment of bronchial asthma. *J Asthma.* (1985); 22: 45–55.

McKeever T.M., Scrivener S., Broadfield E., et al. Prospective study of diet and decline in lung function in a general population. *Am J Respir Crit Care Med.* (2002); 165: 1299–303.

Neuman I., Nahum H., Ben-Amotz A. Reduction of exercise-induced asthma oxidative stress by lycopene, a natural antioxidant. *Allergy.* (2000 Dec); 55(12): 1184–9.

Shaheen S.O., Sterne J.A., Thompson R.L., et al. Dietary antioxidants and asthma in adults: population-based case-control study. *Am J Respir Crit Care Med.* (2001); 164: 1823–8.

Bladder infection (cystitis):

Avorn J., Monane M., Gurwitz J.H., et al. Reduction of bacteriuria and pyuria after ingestion of cranberry juice. *JAMA.* (1994); 271: 751–4.

Guay D.R. Cranberry and urinary tract infections. *Drugs.* (2009); 69: 775–807.

Sobota A.E. Inhibition of bacterial adherence by cranberry juice: potential use for the treatment of urinary tract infections. *J Urol.* (1984); 131: 1013–16.

Constipation:

Attaluri A., Donahoe R., Valestin J., Brown K., Rao S.S. Randomised clinical trial: dried plums (prunes) vs. psyllium for constipation. *Aliment Pharmacol Ther.* (2011 Apr); 33(7): 822–8.

Iacono G., Cavataio F., Montalto G., Florena A., Tumminello M., Soresi M., Notarbartolo A., Carroccio A. Intolerance of cow's milk and chronic constipation in children. *N Engl J Med.* (1998); 339(16): 1100–4.

Lever E., Cole J., Scott S.M., Emery P.W., Whelan K. Systematic review: the effect of prunes on gastrointestinal function. *Aliment Pharmacol Ther.* (2014 Oct); 40(7): 750–8.

Suares N.C., Ford A.C. Systematic review: the effects of fibre in the management of chronic idiopathic constipation. *Aliment Pharmacol Ther.* (2011 Apr); 33(8): 895–901.

Depression:

Christensen L. Psychological distress and diet—effects of sucrose and caffeine. *J Appl Nutr.* (1988); 40: 44–50.

Freeman M.P., Rapaport M.H. Omega-3 fatty acids and depression: from cellular mechanisms to clinical care. *J Clin Psychiatry.* (2011 Feb); 72(2): 258–9.

Ginty A.T., Conklin S.M. Short-term supplementation of acute long-chain omega-3 polyunsaturated fatty acids may alter depression status and decrease symptomology among young adults with depression: a preliminary randomized and placebo controlled trial. *Psychiatry Res.* (2015 Sep 30); 229(1-2): 485–9.

Greden J., Fontaine P., Lubetsky M., et al. Anxiety and depression associated with caffeinism among psychiatric inpatients. *Am J Psychiatry.* (1978); 135: 963–6.

Liu X., Yan Y., Li F., Zhang D. Fruit and vegetable consumption and the risk of depression: a meta-analysis. *Nutrition.* (2016 Mar); 32(3): 296–302.

Onyike C.U., Crum R.M., Lee H.B., et al. Is obesity associated with major depression? Results from the Third National Health and Nutrition Examination Survey. *Am J Epidemiol.* (2003); 158: 1139–47.

Sánchez-Villegas A., Delgado-Rodríguez M., Alonso A., et al. Association of the Mediterranean dietary pattern with the incidence of depression. *Archives Gen Psych.* (2009); 66(10): 1090–8.

Westover A.N., Marangell L.B. A cross-national relationship between sugar consumption and major depression? *Depress Anxiety.* (2002); 16: 118–20.

Winokur A., Maislin G., Phillips J.L., et al. Insulin resistance after oral glucose tolerance testing in patients with major depression. *Am J Psychiatry*. (1988); 145: 325–30.

Diabetes, type 2:

Sargeant L.A., Khaw K.T., Bingham S., et al. Fruit and vegetable intake and population glycosylated haemoglobin levels: the EPIC-Norfolk Study. *Eur J Clin Nutr*. (2001); 55: 342–8.

Williams D.E., Wareham N.J., Cox B.D., et al. Frequent salad vegetable consumption is associated with a reduction in the risk of diabetes mellitus. *J Clin Epidemiol*. (1999); 52: 329–35.

Diarrhea:

Leob H., Vandenplas Y., Wursch P., Guesry P. Tannin-rich carob pod for the treatment of acute-onset diarrhea. *J Pediatr Gastroent Nutr*. (1989); 8: 480–5.

Hostettler M., Steffen R., Tschopp A. Efficacy of tolerability of insoluble carob fraction in the treatment of travellers' diarrhea. *J Diarr Dis Res*. (1995); 13: 155–8.

Ear infection (otitis media):

Bellionin P., Cantani A., Salvinelli F. Allergy: a leading role in otitis media with effusion. *Allergol Immunol*. (1987); 15: 205–8.

Hurst D.S. Association of otitis media with effusion and allergy as demonstrated by intradermal skin testing and eosinophil protein levels in both middle ear effusions and mucosal biopsies. *Laryngoscope*. (1996); 106: 1128–37.

McMahan J.T., Calenoff E., Croft D.J., et al. Chronic otitis media with effusion and allergy: modified RAST analysis of 119 cases. *Otol Head Neck Surg*. (1981); 89: 427–31.

Nsouli T.M., Nsouli S.M., Linde R.E., et al. Role of food allergy in serous otitis media. *Ann Allergy*. (1994); 73: 215–19.

Uhari M., Kontiokari T., Niemela M. A novel use of xylitol sugar in preventing acute otitis media. *Pediatrics*. (1998); 102: 879–84.

Uhari M., Kontiokari T., Koskela M., et al. Xylitol chewing gum in prevention of acute otitis media: double blind randomised trial. *BMJ*. (1996); 313: 1180–4.

Eczema:

Atherton D.J. Role of diet in treating atopic eczema: elimination diets can be beneficial. *BMJ*. (1988 Dec 3); 297(6661):1458, 1460.

Berth-Jones J., Graham-Brown R.A. Placebo-controlled trial of essential fatty acid supplementation in atopic dermatitis. *Lancet*. (1993); 341: 1557–60.

de Maat-Bleeker F., Bruijnzeel-Koomen C. Food allergy in adults with atopic dermatitis. *Monogr Allergy*. (1996); 32: 157–63.

Fiocchi A., Sala M., Signoroni P. et al. The efficacy and safety of gamma-linolenic acid in the treatment of infantile atopic dermatitis. *J Int Med Res*. (1994); 22: 24–32.

Sampson H.A., Scanlon S.M. Natural history of food hypersensitivity in children with atopic dermatitis. *J Pediatr*. (1989); 115: 23–7.

Savolainen J., Lammintausta K., Kalimo K., et al. *Candida albicans* and atopic dermatitis. *Clin Exp Allergy*. (1993); 23: 332–9.

Soyland E., Funk J., Rajka G., et al. Dietary supplementation with long-chain n-3 fatty acids in patients with atopic dermatitis. A double-blind, multi-centre study. *Br J Dermatol*. (1994); 130: 757–64.

Takwale A., Tan E., Agarwal S., et al. Efficacy and tolerability of borage oil in adults and children with atopic eczema: randomised, double blind, placebo controlled, parallel group trial. *BMJ*. (2003); 327: 1385.

Van Bever H.P., Docx M., Stevens W.J. Food and food additives in severe atopic dermatitis. *Allergy*. (1989); 44: 588–94.

Fibrocystic breast disease:

Baghurst P.A., Rohan T.E. Dietary fiber and risk of benign proliferative epithelial disorders of the breast. *Int J Cancer*. (1995); 63: 481–85.

Ernster V.L., Mason L., Goodson W.H. III, et al. Effects of caffeine-free diet on benign breast disease. A random trial. *Surgery*. (1982); 91: 263–7.

Lubin F., Ron E., Wax Y., et al. A case-control study of caffeine and methylxanthine in benign breast disease. *JAMA*. (1985); 253: 2388–92.

Marshall J., Graham S., Swanson M. Caffeine consumption and benign breast disease: a case-control comparison. *Am J Public Health*. (1982); 72: 610–12.

Petrakis N.L., King E.B. Cytological abnormalities in nipple aspirates of breast fluid from women with severe constipation. *Lancet*. (1981); 2: 1203–4.

Food Allergy:

Dockhorn R.J., Smith T.C. Use of a chemically defined hypoallergenc diet in the management of patients with suspected food allergy. *Ann Allergy*. (1981); 47: 264–66.

Lomer M.C. Review article: the aetiology, diagnosis, mechanisms and clinical evidence for food intolerance. *Aliment Pharmacol Ther*. (2015 Feb); 41(3): 262–75.

Osterballe M., Hansen T.K., Mortz C.G., Høst A., Bindslev-Jensen C. The prevalence of food hypersensitivity in an unselected population of children and adults. *Pediatr Allergy Immunol*. (2005); 16: 567–73.

Sicherer S., Sampson H. Food allergy. *J Allergy Clin Immunol*. (2006); 117: S470–5.

Skypala I.J., Williams M., Reeves L., Meyer R., Venter C. Sensitivity to food additives, vaso-active amines and salicylates: a review of the evidence. *Clin Transl Allergy*. (2015 Oct 13); 5: 34.

Gallstones:

Baggio G., Pagnan A., Muraca M., et al. Olive-oil-enriched diet. Effect on serum lipoprotein levels and biliary cholesterol saturation. *Am J Clin Nutr*. (1988); 47: 960–4.

Bell G.D., Doran J. Gallstone dissolution in man using an essential oil preparation. *Br Med J*. (1979); 1: 24.

Breneman J.C. Allergy elimination diet as the most effective gallbladder diet. *Ann Allergy*. (1968); 26: 83–7.

Douglas B.R., Jansen J.B., Tham R.T. Coffee stimulation of cholecystokinin release and gallbladder contraction in humans. *Am J Clin Nutr*. (1990); 52: 553–6.

Ellis W.R., Bell G.D. Treatment of biliary duct stones with a terpene preparation. *Br Med J* (Clin Res Ed). (1981); 282: 611.

Gaby A.R. Nutritional approaches to prevention and treatment of gallstones. *Altern Med*. (Rev. 2009 Sep); 14(3): 258–67.

Hordinsky B.Z. Terpenes in the treatment of gallstones. *Minn Med*. (1971); 54: 649–52.

Jonkers I.J., Smelt A.H., Princen H.M., et al. Fish oil increases bile acid synthesis in male patients with hypertriglyceridemia. *J Nutr*. (2006 Apr); 136(4): 987–91.

Leitzmann M.F., Stampfer M.J., Willett W.C., et al. Coffee intake is associated with lower risk of symptomatic gallstone disease in women. *Gastroenterology*. (2002), 123. 1823–30.

Méndez-Sánchez N., González V., Aguayo P., et al. Fish oil (n-3) polyunsaturated fatty acids beneficially affect biliary cholesterol nucleation time in obese women losing weight. *J Nutr*. (2001 Sep); 131(9): 2300–3.

Moerman C.J., Smeets F.W., Kromhout D. Dietary risk factors for clinically diagnosed gallstones in middle-aged men. A 25-year follow-up study (the Zutphen Study). *Ann Epidemiol*. (1994); 4: 248–54.

Pixley F., Wilson D., McPherson K., et al. Effect of vegetarianism on development of gallstones in women. *Br Med J*. (1985); 291: 11–12.

Thornton J.R., Emmett P.M., Heaton K.W. Diet and gall stones: effects of refined and unrefined carbohydrate diets on bile cholesterol saturation and bile acid metabolism. *Gut*. (1983); 24: 2–6.

Tsai C.J., Leitzmann M.F., Willett W.C., Giovannucci E.L. Glycemic load, glycemic index, and carbohydrate intake in relation to risk of cholecystectomy in women. *Gastroenterology*. (2005 Jul); 129(1): 105–12.

Gastroesophageal reflux disease (GERD) and nonulcer dyspepsia (NUD):

Greally P., Hampton F.J., MacFadyen U.M., Simpson H. Gaviscon and Carobel compared with cisapride in gastroesophageal reflux. *Arch Dis Child*. (1992); 67: 618–21.

Sun J. D-limonene: safety and clinical applications. *Altern Med Rev*. (2007 Sep); 12(3): 259–64.

Yasawy M.I., Randhawa M.A. GERD is becoming a challenge for the medical profession: is there any remedy? *Hepatogastroenterology.* (2014 Sep); 61(134): 1623–6.

Heart disease, atherosclerosis, and high cholesterol levels:

Alvarez-Suarez J.M., Giampieri F., Tulipani S., et al. One-month strawberry-rich anthocyanin supplementation ameliorates cardiovascular risk, oxidative stress markers and platelet activation in humans. *J Nutr Biochem.* (2014 Mar); 25(3): 289–94.

Anderson J.W., Johnstone B.M., Cook-Newell M.E. Meta-analysis of the effects of soy protein intake on serum lipids. *N Engl J Med.* (1995); 333: 276–82.

Chai S.C., Hooshmand S., Saadat R.L., et al. Daily apple versus dried plum: impact on cardiovascular disease risk factors in postmenopausal women. *J Acad Nutr Diet.* (2012 Aug); 112(8): 1158–68.

Gigleux I., Jenkins D.J., Kendall C.W., et al. Comparison of a dietary portfolio diet of cholesterol-lowering foods and a statin on LDL particle size phenotype in hypercholesterolaemic participants. *Br J Nutr.* (2007 Dec); 98(6): 1229–36.

Hyson D.A. A comprehensive review of apples and apple components and their relationship to human health. *Adv Nutr.* (2011 Sep); 2(5): 408–20.

Jenkins D.J., Kendall C.W., Marchie A., et al. Effects of a dietary portfolio of cholesterol-lowering foods vs lovastatin on serum lipids and C-reactive protein. *JAMA.* (2003); 290: 502–10.

Jenkins D.J., Kendall C.W., Faulkner D.A., et al. Long-term effects of a plant-based dietary portfolio of cholesterol-lowering foods on blood pressure. *Eur J Clin Nutr.* (2008 Jun); 62(6): 781–8.

Jorge P.A., Neyra L.C., Osaki R.M., et al. Effect of eggplant on plasma lipid levels, lipidic peroxidation and reversion of endothelial dysfunction in experimental hypercholesterolemia. *Arq Bras Cardiol.* (1998); 70(2): 87–91.

Reynolds K., Chin A., Lees K.A., Nguyen A., Bujnowski D., He J. A meta-analysis of the effect of soy protein supplementation on serum lipids. *Am J Cardiol.* (2006); 98(5): 633–40.

Sable-Amplis R., Sicart R., Agid R. Further studies on the cholesterol-lowering effect of apple in humans. Biochemical mechanisms involved. *Nutr Res.* (1983); 3: 325–83.

Shen J., Wilmot K.A., Ghasemzadeh N., et al. Mediterranean dietary patterns and cardiovascular health. *Annu Rev Nutr.* (2015); 35: 425–49.

Hemorrhoids:

Alonso-Coello P., Mills E., Heels-Ansdell D., López-Yarto M. Fiber for the treatment of hemorrhoids complications: a systematic review and meta-analysis. *Am J Gastroenterol.* (2006 Jan); 101(1): 181–8.

Herpes simplex:

Griffith R., DeLong D.C., Nelson J.D. Relation of arginine-lysine antagonism to herpes simplex growth in tissue culture. *Chemotherapy.* (1981); 27: 209–13.

Griffith R.S., Walsh D.E., Myrmel K.H., et al. Success of L-lysine therapy in frequently recurrent herpes simplex infection. *Dermatologica.* (1987); 175: 183–90.

High blood pressure:

Johnson S.A., Figueroa A., Navaei N., et al. Daily blueberry consumption improves blood pressure and arterial stiffness in postmenopausal women with pre- and stage 1-hypertension: a randomized, double-blind, placebo-controlled clinical trial. *J Acad Nutr Diet.* (2015 Jan 2). pii: S2212-2672(14)01633-5.

Le Q.T. and Elliott W.J. Dose-response relationship of blood pressure and serum cholesterol to 3-n-butylphthalide, a component of celery oil. *Clin Res.* (1991); 39: 750A.

Moore T.J., Vollmer W.M., Appel L.J., et al. Effect of dietary patterns on ambulatory blood pressure : results from the Dietary Approaches to Stop Hypertension (DASH) trial. DASH Collaborative Research Group. *Hypertension.* (1999 Sep); 34(3): 472–7.

Park E., Edirisinghe I., Choy Y.Y., Waterhouse A., Burton-Freeman B. Effects of grape seed extract beverage on blood pressure and metabolic indices in individuals with pre-hypertension: a randomised, double-blinded, two-arm, parallel, placebo-controlled trial. *Br J Nutr*. (2015); Nov 16: 1–13.

Sacks F.M., Svetkey L.P., Vollmer W.M., et al. Effects on blood pressure of reduced dietary sodium and the Dietary Approaches to Stop Hypertension (DASH) diet. DASH–Sodium Collaborative Research Group. *N Engl J Med*. (2001); 344: 3–10.

Hives (urticaria):

Collins-Williams C. Clinical spectrum of adverse reactions to tartrazine. *J Asthma*. (1985); 22: 139–43.

Kulczycki A. Aspartame-induced urticaria. *Ann Intern Med*. (1986); 104: 207–8.

Lessof M.H. Reactions to food additives. *Clin Exp Allergy*. (1995); 25(Suppl 1): 27–8.

Ormerod A.D., Reid T.M., Main R.A. Penicillin in milk—its importance in urticaria. *Clin Allergy*. (1987); 17: 229–34.

Swain A.R., Dutton S.P., Truswell A.S. Salicylates in foods. *J Am Diet Assoc*. (1985); 85: 950–60.

Zuberbier T., Chantraine-Hess S., Hartmann K., et al. Pseudoallergen-free diet in the treatment of chronic urticaria. A prospective study. *Acta Derm Venereol* (Stockh). (1995); 75: 484–7.

Immune support:

Bernstein J., Alpert S., Nauss K., Suskind R. Depression of lymphocyte transformation following oral glucose ingestion. *Am J Clin Nutr*. (1977); 7; 30: 613.

Sanchez A., Reeser J., Lau H., et al. Role of sugars in human neutrophilic phagocytosis. *Am J Clin Nutr*. (1973); 26: 1180–4.

Irritable bowel syndrome (IBS):

Chey W.D. Food: The main course to wellness and illness in patients with irritable bowel syndrome. *Am J Gastroenterol*. (2016 Mar); 111(3): 366–71.

Drisko J., Bischoff B., Hall M., McCallum R. Treating irritable bowel syndrome with a food elimination diet followed by food challenge and probiotics. *J Am Coll Nutr.* (2006 Dec); 25(6): 514–22.

El-Salhy M., Gundersen D. Diet in irritable bowel syndrome. *Nutr J.* (2015 Apr 14); 14: 36.

Eswaran S., Tack J., Chey W.D. Food: the forgotten factor in the irritable bowel syndrome. *Gastroenterol Clin North Am.* (2011 Mar); 40(1): 141–62.

Gertner D., Powell-Tuck J. Irritable bowel syndrome and food intolerance. *Practitioner.* (1994); 238: 499–504.

Mansueto P., D'Alcamo A., Seidita A., Carroccio A. Food allergy in irritable bowel syndrome: the case of non-celiac wheat sensitivity. *World J Gastroenterol.* (2015 Jun 21); 21(23): 7089–109.

Russo A., Fraser R., Horowitz M. The effect of acute hyperglycemia on small intestinal motility in normal subjects. *Diabetologia.* (1996); 39: 984–9.

Shepherd S.J., Parker F.C., Muir J.G., et al. Dietary triggers of abdominal symptoms in patients with irritable bowel syndrome: randomised, placebo-controlled evidence. *Clin Gastroenterol Hepatol.* (2008); 6: 765–71.

Kidney stones:

Borghi L., Meschi T., Amato F., Briganti A., Novarini A., Giannini A. Urinary volume, water and recurrences in idiopathic calcium nephrolithiasis: a 5-year randomized prospective study. *J Urol.* (1996); 155: 839–43.

Friedlander J.I., Antonelli J.A., Pearle M.S. Diet: from food to stone. *World J Urol.* (2015 Feb); 33(2): 179–85. doi:10.1007/s00345-014-1344-z.

Nouvenne A., Meschi T., Prati B., et al. Effects of low salt diet on idiopathic hypercalciuria in calcium oxalate stone formers: a 3-mo randomized controlled trial. *Am J Clin Nutr.* (2010); 91: 565–70.

Robertson W., Peacock M., Marshall D. Prevalence of urinary stone disease in vegetarians. *Eur Urol.* (1982); 8: 334–9.

Shuster J., Jenkins A., Logan C., et al. Soft drink consumption and urinary stone recurrence: a randomized prevention trial. *J Clin Epidemiol.* (1992); 45: 911–16.

Siener R., Hesse A. The effect of a vegetarian and different omnivorous diets on urinary risk factors for uric acid stone formation. *Eur J Nutr*. (2003); 42: 332–7.

Taylor E.N., Curhan G.C. Diet and fluid prescription in stone disease. *Kidney Int*. (2006 Sep); 70(5): 835–9.

Thom J., Morris J., Bishop A., et al. The influence of refined carbohydrate on urinary calcium excretion. *Br J Urol*. (1978); 50: 459–64.

Macular degeneration:

Carpentier S., Knaus M., Suh M. Associations between lutein, zeaxanthin, and age-related macular degeneration: an overview. *Crit Rev Food Sci Nutr*. (2009 Apr); 49(4): 313–26.

SanGiovanni J.P., Agrón E., Clemons T.E., Chew E.Y. Omega-3 long-chain polyunsaturated fatty acid intake inversely associated with 12-year progression to advanced age-related macular degeneration. *Arch Ophthalmol*. (2009 Jan); 127(1): 110–12.

Seddon J.M., Cote J., Rosner B. Progression of age-related macular degeneration: association with dietary fat, transunsaturated fat, nuts, and fish intake. *Arch Ophthalmol*. (2003); 121: 1728–37.

Menopause:

Dew T.P., Williamson G. Controlled flax interventions for the improvement of menopausal symptoms and postmenopausal bone health: a systematic review. *Menopause*. (2013 Nov); 20(11): 1207–15.

Franco O.H., Chowdhury R., Troup J., et al. Use of plant-based therapies and menopausal symptoms: a systematic review and meta-analysis. *JAMA*. (2016 Jun 21); 315(23): 255463.

Kohama T., Negami M. Effect of low-dose French maritime pine bark extract on climacteric syndrome in 170 perimenopausal women: a randomized, double-blind, placebo-controlled trial. *J Reprod Med*. (2013); 58: 39–46.

Migraine headaches:

Carter C.M., Egger J., Soothill J.F. A dietary management of severe childhood migraine. *Hum Nutr Appl Nutr*. (1985); 39: 294–303.

Dexter J.D., Roberts J., Byer J.A. The five hour glucose tolerance test and effect of low sucrose diet in migraine. *Headache.* (1978); 18: 91–4.

Glueck C.J., McCarren T., Hitzemann R., et al. Amelioration of severe migraine with omega-3 fatty acids: a double-blind, placebo-controlled clinical trial. *Am J Clin Nutr.* (1986); 43: 710.

Harel Z., Gascon G., Riggs S., et al. Supplementation with omega-3 polyunsaturated fatty acids in the management of recurrent migraines in adolescents. *J Adolesc Health.* (2002); 31: 154–61.

Mansfield L.E., Vaughan T.R., Waller S.F., et al. Food allergy and adult migraine: double-blind and mediator confirmation of an allergic etiology. *Ann Allergy.* (1985); 55: 126–9.

Mauskop A., Altura B.M. Role of magnesium in the pathogenesis and treatment of migraines. *Clin Neurosci.* (1998); 5: 24–7.

Wilkinson C.F. Jr. Recurrent migrainoid headaches associated with spontaneous hypoglycemia. *Am J Med Sci.* (1949); 218: 209–12.

Osteoarthritis:

Green J.A., Hirst-Jones K.L., Davidson R.K. The potential for dietary factors to prevent or treat osteoarthritis. *Proc Nutr Soc.* (2014 May); 73(2): 278–88.

Lopez H.L. Nutritional interventions to prevent and treat osteoarthritis. Part I: focus on fatty acids and macronutrients. *PMR.* (2012 May); 4(5 Suppl): S145–54.

Shen C.L., Smith B.J., Lo D.F., et al. Dietary polyphenols and mechanisms of osteoarthritis. *J Nutr Biochem.* (2012 Nov); 23(11): 1367–77.

Osteoporosis:

Bartolozzi E. The natural approach to osteoporosis. *Clin Cases Miner Bone Metab.* (2015 May–Aug); 12(2): 111–15.

Hooshmand S., Brisco J.R., Arjmandi B.H. The effect of dried plum on serum levels of receptor activator of NF-k ligand, osteoprotegerin and sclerostin in osteopenic postmenopausal women: a randomised controlled trial. *Br J Nutr.* (2014 Jul 14); 112(1): 55–60.

Knapen M.H., Drummen N.E., Smit E., Vermeer C., Theuwissen E. Three-year low-dose menaquinone-7 supplementation helps decrease bone loss in healthy postmenopausal women. *Osteoporos Int*. (2013); 24(9): 2499–507.

Lagari V.S., Levis S. Phytoestrogens for menopausal bone loss and climacteric symptoms. *J Steroid Biochem Mol Biol*. (2014 Jan); 139: 294–301.

Rizzoli R. Nutritional aspects of bone health. *Best Pract Res Clin Endocrinol Metab*. (2014 Dec); 28(6): 795–808.

Sacco S.M., Horcajada M.N., Offord E. Phytonutrients for bone health during ageing. *Br J Clin Pharmacol*. (2013 Mar); 75(3): 697–707.

Prostate enlargement (benign prostatic hyperplasia):

Grainger E.M., Hadley C.W., Moran N.E., et al. A comparison of plasma and prostate lycopene in response to typical servings of tomato soup, sauce or juice in men before prostatectomy. *Br J Nutr*. (2015 Aug 28); 114(4): 596–607.

Kucuk O., Sarkar F.H., Sakr W., et al. Phase II randomized clinical trial of lycopene supplementation before radical prostatectomy. *Cancer Epidemiol Biomarkers Prev*. (2001); 10: 861–8.

Vidlar A., Vostalova J., Ulrichova J., et al. The effectiveness of dried cranberries (Vaccinium macrocarpon) in men with lower urinary tract symptoms. *Br J Nutr*. (2010 Oct); 104(8): 1181–9. Epub 2010 Aug 31.

Psoriasis:

Belcaro G., Luzzi R., Hu S., et al. Improvement in signs and symptoms in psoriasis patients with Pycnogenol® supplementation. *Panminerva Med*. (2014); 56(1): 41–8.

Bhatia B.K., Millsop J.W., Debbaneh M., et al. Diet and psoriasis, part II: celiac disease and role of a gluten-free diet. *J Am Acad Dermatol*. (2014 Aug); 71(2): 350–8.

Debbaneh M., Millsop J.W., Bhatia B.K., Koo J., Liao W. Diet and psoriasis, part I: impact of weight loss interventions. *J Am Acad Dermatol*. (2014 Jul); 71(1): 133–40.

Guida B., Napoleone A., Trio R., Nastasi A., Balato N., Laccetti R., Cataldi M. Energy-restricted, n-3 polyunsaturated fatty acids-rich diet improves the clinical response to immuno-modulating drugs in obese patients with plaque-type psoriasis: a randomized control clinical trial. *Clin Nutr.* (2014 Jun); *33*(3): 399–405.

Millsop J.W., Bhatia B.K., Debbaneh M., Koo J., Liao W. Diet and psoriasis, part III: role of nutritional supplements. *J Am Acad Dermatol.* (2014 Sep); *71*(3): 561–9.

Rheumatoid arthritis:

Darlington L.G., Ramsey N.W. Clinical review. Review of dietary therapy for rheumatoid arthritis. *Br J Rheumatol.* 1(993); *32*: 507–14.

Kjeldsen-Kragh J. Rheumatoid arthritis treated with vegetarian diets. *Am J Clin Nutr.* (1999); 70(Suppl): 594S–600S.

Kjeldsen-Kragh J., Haugen M., Borchgrevink C.F., et al. Controlled trial of fasting and one-year vegetarian diet in rheumatoid arthritis. *Lancet.* (1991); *338*: 899–902.

Ulcer:

Cheney G. Anti-peptic ulcer dietary factor. *J Am Diet Assoc.* (1950); 26: 668–72.

Cheney G. Rapid healing of peptic ulcers in patients receiving fresh cabbage juice. *Cal Med.* (1949); 70: 10–14.

Kang J.Y., Tay H.H., Guan R., et al. Dietary supplementation with pectin in the maintenance treatment of duodenal ulcer. A controlled study. *Scand J Gastroenterol.* (1988); 23: 95–9.

Kumar N., Kumar A., Broor S.L., et al. Effect of milk on patients with duodenal ulcers. *Br Med J.* (1986); 293: 666.

Rydning A., Berstad A., Aadland E., et al. Prophylactic effect of dietary fiber in duodenal ulcer disease. *Lancet.* (1982); 2: 736–9.

Yanaka A., Fahey J.W., Fukumoto A., et al. Dietary sulforaphane-rich broccoli sprouts reduce colonization and attenuate gastritis in *Helicobacter pylori*-infected mice and humans. *Cancer Prev Res* (Phila). (2009 Apr); 2(4): 353–60.

Varicose veins:

Cesarone M.R., Belcaro G., Rohdewald P., et al. Improvement of signs and symptoms of chronic venous insufficiency and microangiopathy with Pycnogenol: a prospective, controlled study. *Phytomedicine.* (2010 Sep); 17(11): 835–9.

Gulati O.P. Pycnogenol® in chronic venous insufficiency and related venous disorders. *Phytother Res.* (2014 Mar); 28(3): 348–62.

Visudhiphan S., Poolsuppasit S., Piboonnukarintr O., Tumliang S. The relationship between high fibrinolytic activity and daily capsicum ingestion in Thais. *Am J Clin Nutr.* (1982); 35: 1452–8.

Index

About the Author

Dr. Michael T. Murray is the author of more than thirty books, including the acclaimed bestsellers *The Encyclopedia of Natural Medicine* (Third Edition) and *The Encyclopedia of Healing Foods* (coauthored with Dr. Joseph Pizzorno). He is regarded as the world authority on natural medicine and appears regularly in national media, including *The Dr. Oz Show*. An educator, lecturer, researcher, and health food industry consultant, Dr. Murray also constantly updates his health information portal: DoctorMurray.com.